Clinical Thinking in Psychotherapy

Clinical Thinking in Psychotherapy empowers practitioners and students to better understand clients by attending to both verbal and nonverbal forms of expression. Readers will find tools for unlearning biases and for providing effective therapy with transcripts and dialogic tools.

Chapters focus on how to practice clinical thinking, how to teach it, and how to reflect on what is being taught. Therapists, supervisors, and students alike will come away from this book with decision tree questions and prompts, as well as metacognitive questions for structuring consultations and producing desirable outcomes for the clinician and the patient.

Jon Frederickson, MSW, faculty of the New Washington School of Psychiatry, has written over fifty published papers, seven books, and numerous skill-building exercises designed for therapists.

This groundbreaking book brilliantly bridges the gap between theoretical understanding and practical application. The trans-theoretical text will help clinicians training in a broad range of psychotherapy models. Numerous transcripts show how to develop therapists' clinical acumen. A must-read for anyone striving to excel in the art and science of psychotherapy.

Tony Rousmaniere, PsyD, *program director, Sentio University, and president, Division 29 of the American Psychological Association (Society for the Advancement of Psychotherapy)*

This multifaceted gem of a book is a masterpiece. Detailed process recordings showcase scientific inquiry between student and teacher—collaborative conversations that show how to translate clinical thinking into embodied practice. It is destined to become a classic in the field of psychotherapy training and supervision.

Martha Stark, MD, *faculty, Harvard Medical School*

Clinical thinking calls upon cognition, emotion, memory, perception, and behavior, in an integration not easily described. Fredrickson has systematically demystified this process, with generous verbatim examples of how he teaches. Firmly anchored in science, the book is a fine guide to mastering a daunting art. I recommend it enthusiastically to all students, practitioners, supervisors, and teachers of psychotherapy.

Nancy McWilliams, PhD, ABPP, *visiting professor emerita, Rutgers Graduate School of Applied and Professional Psychology*

Clinical Thinking in Psychotherapy

What It Is, How It Works, and
Why and How to Teach It

Jon Frederickson

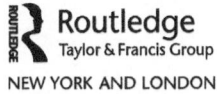

Routledge
Taylor & Francis Group

NEW YORK AND LONDON

Designed cover image: © Quickshooting @Getty Images

First published 2025
by Routledge
605 Third Avenue, New York, NY 10158

and by Routledge
4 Park Square, Milton Park, Abingdon, Oxon, OX14 4RN

Routledge is an imprint of the Taylor & Francis Group, an informa business

© 2025 Jon Frederickson

ISBN: 978-1-032-77764-1 (hbk)
ISBN: 978-1-032-77757-3 (pbk)
ISBN: 978-1-003-48863-7 (ebk)

DOI: 10.4324/9781003488637

Typeset in Sabon
by SPi Technologies India Pvt Ltd (Straive)

For Product Safety Concerns and Information please contact our EU representative: GPSR@taylorandfrancis.com
Taylor & Francis Verlag GmbH, Kaufingerstraße 24, 80331 München, Germany

Contents

Acknowledgments

I'd like to thank Sanne Almeborg, Lars Brusell, F. Barton Evans, Allan Gold, Bill Gottdiener, Maury Joseph, Nat Kuhn, Nicole Lediard, Peter Liliengren, Tom Marup, Teri Scott, Everett Siegel, Alessandro Talia, and Irv Weiner for their comments on previous drafts of this book. Special thanks are due to Diane Byster and Bjorn Elwin, whose criticisms, editing, and support greatly improved the organization and clarity of the book. I am most grateful to Hope Hartman, whose extensive comments added immensely to the sections involving metacognitive knowledge. And, finally, I would like to thank my colleagues at the Washington School of Psychiatry with whom we founded a supervision training program over thirty years ago. Our work together set me off on a journey that led to this book. I would also like to express my gratitude to Sarah Pillsbury, Michael Stadter, Irv Schneider, Bernardo Hirschman, Gerry Perman, Gordon Kirschner, Monroe Pray, Jack Love, Harold Eist, Habib Davanloo, and Patricia Coughlin, supervisors whose work inspires me to this day. And I would like to thank all the patients, supervisees, and students I have worked with over the years who kept teaching me what I am still learning: how to think clinically.

Chapter 1

Why We Teach Clinical Thinking in Psychotherapy

Jon Frederickson

What do we want students to learn when we teach or supervise psychotherapy? Do we want them to memorize facts, concepts, theories, and techniques? Yes. But to what purpose? So students can think clinically to intervene effectively and save lives.

In any field, to know what to do, we need to know what is going on. To solve a problem, we try to understand it. And, to understand a problem, we think about it. Good thinking leads to effective actions, whether you are a surgeon, a chess master, or a therapist. In psychotherapy, therapists engage in clinical thinking to diagnose what causes patients' psychological problems. Then, they can treat the cause.

The instructor begins by teaching students how to use concepts to analyze the patient's words and deeds. Then, they can develop a hypothesis and test it through an intervention. Next, the instructor teaches how to assess whether the patient's response confirms the hypothesis. As a result, students can think about their thinking, revise it, and intervene more effectively. They learn how to learn from the patient.

Numerous studies have documented the effectiveness of psychotherapy (Wampold & Imel, 2015). Some therapists are so impressive that researchers call them "super shrinks" (Ricks, 1974). In fact, 20% of clinicians are more effective than the other 80% combined (Miller & Hubble, 2011). But, in other studies, 38% of therapists are consistently unhelpful (Kraus et al., 2011). Why?

On average, graduate school education does not improve trainees' outcomes (Nyman, Nafziger, & Smith, 2011). In one study, 76% of experienced therapists said they lack the skill to motivate patients to work hard in therapy (Orlinsky & Ronnstad, 2005). Moreover, less than 47% felt a sense of mastery. So, while therapy can be effective, psychotherapy training often is not.

When graduate education does not help therapists become effective, what about supervision? According to Ellis et al. (2014), 93% of supervision is inadequate and 35% harmful. Moreover, many supervisors practice

DOI: 10.4324/9781003488637-1

incompetently (Binder, 1993; Milne & James, 2002). Why? They "typically receive little to no training in how to ... do supervision" (Watkins, 1998). No wonder a recent meta-analysis showed supervision contributed less than 1% to patient outcomes (Whipple et al., 2020). Even so, both supervisors and students want to be effective.

How do these training problems affect therapists' ability to assess their skill level and learning needs? In one study, the median therapist ranked himself in the 80th percentile (Walfish et al., 2012). None ranked themselves below the 75th percentile. Apparently, therapists are not learning to think about their thinking and interventions. Otherwise, they would not assess themselves so inaccurately. In another study, therapists predicted fewer than 5% of patients' deteriorations (Hannan et al., 2005). Which ones were best at predicting the cases that would deteriorate? Graduate students! Does our capacity for self-appraisal become worse with experience? Several studies suggest this is the case (Ægisdóttir et al., 2006). Further, didactic continuing education programs do not improve patient outcomes. Why? They do not emphasize skill development (Taylor & Neimeyer, 2017). Perhaps this explains why therapists become less effective over time (Goldberg et al., 2016).

Yet teachers and supervisors work hard to help students reach their potential. Therapists continue to seek skills through training, supervision, and conferences. So why does psychotherapy education help a few students but fail so many others? Does the fault lie with students and supervisors? Or could we reconceive the purpose of psychotherapy training and supervision and how we do it?

The literature has suggested many causes for these problems. For instance, most supervisors "receive minimal training in supervision skills" (Spence et al., 2001, p. 151). However, Watkins & Scaturo (2014) make a more fundamental criticism: with a few exceptions (Gordan, 1997; James, 2006; Szecsody, 1997), research in learning, memory, and teaching does not guide most psychotherapy teaching or supervision (Scaturo & Watkins, 2014).

Learning sciences literature shows that every complex body of knowledge has a theory that guides the thinking in that field. The theory and concepts we use are called declarative knowledge. And we translate theory into practice through techniques and interventions—procedural knowledge. Conditional knowledge tells us when, where, and why we use those interventions. And metacognitive knowledge results when we analyze what patients' responses are teaching us so that we can improve and refine our thinking.

Now, we can analyze psychotherapy education from the perspective of learning sciences research. Sometimes, students learn a theory (declarative knowledge) but not how to apply it in practice (procedural knowledge). For instance, they can define "defense" but not identify or address one in a session. A recent graduate course taught eight theories in one semester but not how to apply them. In such a class, theory appears to be an irrelevant abstraction because students do not learn to use a theory to think clinically and intervene effectively.

Some students learn techniques but not how to use clinical concepts for clinical thinking (declarative knowledge). Thus, clinical reasoning cannot guide their interventions. Students learn techniques but not when or why to use them or with whom (conditional knowledge). Then, guessing or imitating determines when they intervene. Or they rely on a few techniques, leading to ritualism and stereotypy (Peterfreund, 2019). This results from the "McDonaldization of teaching" (Pearson, 2007, p. 154), when instructors teach routine techniques but not higher-order thinking skills.

As a result, some students do not learn how to assess if their interventions helped the patient. They do not know how to think about their thinking to improve it. No wonder the average therapist believes she is in the top 20%! She did not learn to hear the patient's supervision—metacognitive knowledge.

Psychotherapy always involves knowledge of a psychological theory and how to apply it in practice. However, some students learn theory but not technique. Others learn techniques but not how to use a theory for clinical thinking. As a result, they do not know when to intervene, with whom, and why. So, let's turn to a possible solution to these common educational problems.

Teaching and supervising psychotherapy is an extraordinarily complex task, described in a vast literature. (See, e.g., Alonso & Rutan, 1988; Benedek & Fleming, 1983; Dewald, 1987; Ekstein & Wallerstein, 1972; Jacobs, David, & Meyer, 1997; McWilliams, 2021; Watkins, 2014.) But this task has a primary goal: to teach students how to think clinically to intervene effectively. Therefore, this book will focus on how to do clinical thinking and how to teach it by integrating research from the learning sciences.

We will begin by describing clinical thinking in psychotherapy. To learn clinical thinking with psychological concepts, however, students must let go of the assumptions and biases in their pre-existing folk psychology. Everyone needs to understand people. And each subculture or class has a folk psychology for doing so. Thus, students often rely on unconscious assumptions for unscientific forms of thinking. So, we help students shift from implicit preconceptions so that they can use explicit psychological concepts for clinical thinking. Likewise, every social group has story-telling strategies for describing people's problems (Churchland, 1998; Ratcliffe, 2007). Therefore, we help students shift from their former descriptions based on unconscious assumptions. Then, they can use psychological concepts for case formulations. And in contrast to folk psychology, they analyze patients' responses to revise their thinking.

Students unlearn old biases and experience the limits of their prior assumptions. Their usual listening approach proves to be inadequate. So they learn new listening skills. When students change how they think, talk, listen, and relate, they change as persons. As a result, anxiety rises. Therefore, teachers help regulate students' anxiety. Otherwise, they will revert to their former layperson styles of thinking and listening.

As students let go of their folk concepts, they learn four kinds of knowledge in psychotherapy training. Those are declarative, procedural, conditional, and metacognitive knowledge (Anderson & Krathwohl, 2001; Pintrich, 2002). Each requires a different form of instruction. Transcripts will illustrate these types of knowledge and how to teach them. Research on the learning sciences, cognitive science, and memory will provide us with a new integrative model for teaching clinical thinking.

I will use psychodynamic theory to illustrate the principles for teaching clinical thinking. However, these principles of teaching and learning apply to any treatment model based on a comprehensive psychological theory, for example cognitive/behavioral therapy (Hofman, Hayes, & Lorscheid, 2021).

We must link clinical thinking to effective therapeutic action. Why is it necessary to look at theories about learning and teaching? What we think students need to learn and how we think they learn affects what and how we teach them (Thayer-Bacon, 1997). So, to begin, let's define what clinical thinking is in psychotherapy.

References

Ægisdóttir, S., White, M., Spengler, P., Maugherman, A., Anderson, R., Cook, L., Rush, J. (2006). The meta-analysis of clinical judgment project: Fifty-six years of accumulated research on clinical versus statistical prediction. *The Counseling Psychologist, 34*, 341–382.

Alonso, A., & Rutan, S. (1988). Shame and guilt in supervision. *Psychotherapy Theory, Research, and Practice, 25*(4), 576–581. https://doi.org/10.1037/h0085384

Anderson, L. W., & Krathwohl, D. R. (2001). *A taxonomy* for learning, teaching, and assessing: *A revision of Bloom's taxonomy of educational objectives* (abridged ed.). Boston, Mass.: Allyn and Bacon.

Benedek, T., & Fleming, J. (1983). *Psychoanalytic supervision: A model of clinical training*. New York: International Universities Press.

Binder, J. (1993). Is it time to improve psychotherapy training? *Clinical Psychology Review, 13*, 301–318.

Churchland, P. M. (1998). Folk psychology. In P. M. Churchland and P. S. Churchland, *On the contrary: critical essays 1987–1997* (pp. 3–16). Cambridge, Mass.: MIT Press.

Dewald, P. (1987). *Learning process in psychoanalytic supervision: Challenges and complexities*. Madison, Conn.: International Universities Press.

Ekstein, R., & Wallerstein, R. (1972). *The teaching and learning of psychotherapy* (2nd ed.). New York: International Universities Press.

Ellis, M. V., Berger, L., Hanus, A. E., Ayala, E. E., Swords, B. A., & Siembor, M. (2014). Inadequate and harmful clinical supervision: Testing a revised framework and assessing occurrence. *The Counseling Psychologist, 42*(4), 434–472.

Facione, N., & Facione, P. (2008). *Critical thinking and clinical reasoning in the health sciences: An international multidisciplinary teaching anthology.* Millbrae, Ca.: California Academic Press.

Goldberg, S. B., Rousmaniere, T., Miller, S. D., Whipple, J., Nielsen, S. L., Hoyt, W. T., & Wampold, B. E. (2016). Do psychotherapists improve with time and experience? A longitudinal analysis of outcomes in a clinical setting. *Journal of Counseling Psychology, 63*(1), 1–11.

Gordan, K. (1997). An advanced training in the supervision and teaching of psychotherapy. In B. Martindale, M. Morner, M. Rodriguez, & J. Vidit (Eds.), *Supervision and its vicissitudes* (pp. 135–146). London: Karnac.

Hannan, C., Lambert, M., Harmon, C., Nielsen, S., Smart, D., Shimokawa, K., & Scott, W. (2005). A lab test and algorithms for identifying clients at risk for treatment failure. *Journal of Clinical Psychology, 61*(2), 155–163.

Hofman, S., Hayes, S., & Lorscheid, D. (2021). *Learning process-based therapy: A skills training manual for targeting the core processes of psychological change in clinical practice.* Oakland, Ca.: Context Press.

Jacobs, D., David, P., & Meyer, D. (1997). *The supervisory encounter: A guide for teachers of psychodynamic psychotherapy and psychoanalysis.* New Haven, Conn.: Yale University Press.

James, I., Milne, D., Marie-Blackburn, I., & Armstrong, P. (2006). Conducting successful supervision: Novel elements towards an integrative approach. *Behavioural and Cognitive Psychotherapy, 35,* 191–200. https://doi.org/10.1017/S1352465806003407

Kraus, D., Castonguay, L., Nordberg, S., & Hayes, J. (2011). Therapist effectiveness: Implications for accountability and patient care. *Psychotherapy Research, 21*(3), 267–276.

McWilliams, N. (2021). *Psychoanalytic supervision.* New York: Guilford Press.

Miller, S., & Hubble, M. (2011). The road to mastery. *Psychotherapy Networker, 32,* 22–60.

Milne, D., & James, I. (2002). The observed impact of training on competence in clinical supervision. *British Journal of Clinical Psychology, 41,* 55–72.

Nyman, S. J., Nafziger, M. A., & Smith, T. B. (2011). Client outcomes across counselor training level with a multi-tiered supervision model. *Journal of Counseling and Development, 88,* 204–209.

Orlinsky, D., & Ronnstad, M. (2005). *How psychotherapists develop: Therapeutic work and professional development.* Washington, D.C.: American Psychological Association.

Pearson, P. (2007). An endangered species act for literacy education. *Journal of Literacy Research, 39,* 145–162.

Peterfreund, E. (2019). *The process of psychoanalytic therapy.* New York: Routledge.

Pintrich, P. (2002). The role of metacognitive knowledge in teaching, learning, and assessing. *Theory into Practice, 41*(4), 219–225.

Ratcliffe, M. (2007). *Rethinking commonsense psychology: A critique of folk psychology, theory of mind and simulation*. London: Palgrave MacMillan.

Ricks, D. (1974). Supershrink: Methods of a therapist judged successful on the basis of adult outcomes of adolescent patients. In D. F. Ricks, A. Thomas, & M. Roff (Eds.), *Life history research in psychopathology (Vol. 3)*. Minneapolis: University of Minnesota Press.

Rush, D. (2009). The meta-analysis of clinical judgment project: Effects of experience on judgement accuracy. *The Counseling Psychologist, 37*, 350–399.

Scaturo, J., & Watkins, C. (2014). Supervising integrative and eclectic psychotherapies. In C. E. Watkins, Jr. & D. L. Milne (Eds.), *The Wiley international handbook of clinical supervision* (pp. 552–575). New York: Wiley-Blackwell.

Spence, S., Wilson, J., Kavanaugh, D., Strong, J., Murchoch, B., & Krasny, J. (2001). Supervision practices in the allied mental health professions: A review of the evidence. *Behavior Change, 18*, 135–155.

Szecsody, I. (1997). How is learning possible in psychoanalytic supervision? *Psychoanalytic Inquiry, 28*, 373–386.

Taylor, J., & Neimeyer, G. (2017). The ongoing evolution of continuing education: Past, present, and future. In T. Rousmaniere, R. Goodyear, S. Miller, & B. Wampold (Eds.), *The cycle of excellence: Using deliberate practice to improve supervision and training* (pp. 219–238). New York: Wiley.

Thayer-Bacon, B. (1997). The nurturing of a relational epistemology. *Educational Theory, 47*(2), 239–260.

Walfish, S., McAlister, B., O'Donnell, P., & Lambert, M. J. (2012). An investigation of self-assessment bias in mental health providers. *Psychological Reports, 110*(2), 639–644. https://doi.org/10.2466/02.07.17.PR0.110.2.2

Wampold, B., & Imel, Z. (2015). *The great psychotherapy debate: The evidence for what makes psychotherapy work* (2nd ed.).New York: Routledge.

Watkins, C. (1998). Psychotherapy supervision in the 21st century: Some pressing needs and impressing possibilities. *The Journal for Psychotherapy Supervision and Practice, 7*(2), 93–101.

Watkins, C. (2014). The competent psychoanalytic supervisor: Some thoughts about supervisory competencies for accountable practice and training. *International Form for Psychoanalysis, 23*(4), 220–228.

Watkins, C., & Scaturo, D. (2014). Proposal for a common language, educationally-informed model of psychoanalytic supervision. *Psychoanalytic Inquiry, 34*, 619–633.

Whipple, J., Swift, J., Rousmaniere, T., Pederson, T. & Worthen, V. (2020). Supervisor variance in psychotherapy outcome in routine practice: A replication. *SAGE Open, 10*(1). https://doi.org/10.1177/2158244019899047

Chapter 2

What Is Clinical Thinking?

Jon Frederickson

The Elements of Clinical Thinking

"Whenever we think, we think for a purpose within a point of view based on assumptions leading to implications and consequences. We use concepts, ideas, and theories to interpret data, facts, and experiences in order to answer questions, solve problems, and resolve issues" (Hawkins, Elder, & Paul, 2010, p. 5).

No single model of clinical thinking applies across all healthcare specialties. Instead, each specialty has a domain of study, a theory for understanding it, and a unique set of skills (Higgs, 2006). Thus, specialists engage in the form of clinical thinking specific to their field. Yet these different forms of clinical thinking share certain commonalities across disciplines. So, let us examine the elements of clinical thinking (Hawkins, Elder, & Paul, 2010).

1 *The Purpose.* Clinical thinking saves lives by answering this *question*, "What causes this patient's psychological problems?" The therapist ascribes meaning to *data* (a patient shaking) by using *concepts* (anxiety). Then she makes *hypotheses*. ("Perhaps the patient is anxious.") Next, she *tests* a hypothesis through an intervention. ("Are you aware of feeling anxious?") The therapist thinks clinically to discover the cause of patients' psychological suffering. Then, she can treat the cause and reduce patients' symptoms. Better thinking helps us understand patients so that we can offer effective interventions to resolve psychological problems.

2 *A shared point of view.* Therapists recognize the value of biological, psychological, and sociological points of view. But they reason from a *biopsychosocial point of view* (Engel, 1980). They use psychological facts, concepts, hypotheses, and theories. Thus, their thinking has clinical *implications* for treating psychological problems.

DOI: 10.4324/9781003488637-2

The emphasis on biological, sociological, or psychological factors varies among clinicians. For example, those trained in medicine may de-emphasize psychological factors (Rose, 1998) and engage in biological reductionism. Reductionism can also occur when therapists prefer sociological or cultural explanations (DiTomaso, 1982) for psychological problems. Likewise, we can engage in psychological reductionism by ignoring biological or sociological factors (Hayes, 1995). Ideally, we avoid those forms of reductionism by holding an integrative biopsychosocial perspective.

3 *Shared key assumptions provide a basis from which to begin.* Psychotherapists use a theory of psychology to understand psychological problems. And each theory operates with implicit assumptions. For instance, in psychodynamic therapy, we assume defenses cause psychological symptoms. A cognitive-behavioral therapist assumes maladaptive cognitions are the cause. However, we form a new hypothesis when these assumptions prove ineffective. And we assume that we must listen to patients' responses to tailor our work to their needs and capacities.

4 *Shared questions and problems, which we try to solve.* We ask, "What causes this patient's psychological problems and symptoms? Based on the diagnosis of the cause, what interventions do we use?" For instance, a patient describes her doubts about marrying her fiancé and asks, "What do you think I should do?" Thinking clinically, we analyze the function of her question. Did it help her describe her doubts or inhibit her from doing so? Here, her question stopped her from sharing her views. Thus, we can help her see her conflict.

Therapist: You asked for my opinion [*defense*], but a moment ago, you were freer to share your own [*wish*]. Did something feel risky about letting your opinion stand here?

If we can help her see the defense and the fear that triggered it, she may gain greater freedom to offer her views. Her initial problem was a conflict about expressing her opinion. Thus, we could try to solve it by analyzing the function of her question to the therapist (A. Freud, 1936; Davison, Bristol, & Pray, 1986; Davison, Pray, & Bristol, 1990; Gray, 1994). As a result, we can discover the conflicts driving her self-doubt.

5 *Shared information forms the empirical basis for our thinking.* Clinical facts are the basis for our thinking: what the patient says and does and what the therapist says and does in the sessions. For instance, the patient above expressed an opinion. Then she invited the therapist to offer his. Those are two clinical facts.

6 *Shared concepts and ideas help us organize facts into patterns.* We use concepts from a psychological theory to organize data into information. Next, we ask whether this information can be verified or falsified. Further, we analyze how we organize data and the concepts we use. In

contrast, when we use biases or unconscious, unwarranted assumptions, we do not reflect on them or how they shape our perceptions and judgments. Nor do we check whether the information they yield can be verified or falsified.

7   *Shared methods of interpreting data.* Psychotherapists can interpret data through many forms of analysis. Here are some examples:

> We can analyze data through the perspective of *latent content* (Gill & Hoffman, 1983a, 1983b; Langs, 1989a, 1989b). How might the patient's descriptions of other people symbolize how she experiences the therapist?
>
> Or we can interpret data by *analyzing the process* (Gray, 1994). For instance, did this statement help the patient describe her feelings or prevent her from doing so?
>
> Or we can analyze data through the perspective of *enactment* (Levenson, 1972, 1984, 1991; Loewald, 1989). What two roles are the patient and I enacting in therapy? How do these roles parallel the enactment with his wife and boss? How am I perpetuating this enactment? What feelings do I avoid through this enactment? These questions help us analyze data through the perspective of enactment.

8   *Shared methods of metacognition.* Psychotherapists think about their thinking to improve it. Do patients' responses confirm or disconfirm our hypotheses? If not, we revise and retest our hypotheses continually. Then, metacognition improves the quality of our clinical thinking and interventions.

We can question any of these elements to develop and refine our thinking. (See Paul & Elder, 2019, for more on these shared elements.)

But it is not enough to think about a patient's difficulties. After all, our thinking can be, and often is, mistaken. Thus, the student learns to analyze her thinking to improve it and her interventions. To do so, she reflects on how she arrived at her assessment. What evidence did she rely upon to form her hypothesis? What concepts did she use to analyze the patient's words and deeds? What was her listening approach? Did the patient's response to her intervention confirm or disconfirm her hypothesis? How did the patient's feedback change her thinking and hypothesis? Now, thinking about her thinking—metacognition—can guide her reasoning and actions (Facione, 1990).

The therapist uses the patient's feedback to improve her clinical thinking. Otherwise, biases and assumptions lead to non-scientific thinking uninfluenced by the patient's responses. First, we think clinically to understand, diagnose, and treat the patient's symptoms (Facione & Facione, 2008). Next, we analyze the patient's responses to intervention and use that feedback to refine our thinking, hypotheses, and interventions (Facione & Facione, 2008).

In non-scientific thinking, the student does not see her assumptions. In her egocentric thinking, she may treat her assumption as a fact. "If I think it, that makes it so." Since she lacks an empirical approach to assess whether the patient's responses confirm her belief, she cannot systematically use patient feedback to change her thinking and interventions. As in Plato's chariot analogy, the student may imagine she is driving her thoughts (Plato, 2005). But her folk theory—misconceptions, biases, and unconscious assumptions—determines what she can see and think about.

The Role of Theory in Clinical Thinking

Do we need a theory to think about people? Yes. Every person has a theory for understanding others. The question is whether students use a folk theory, unconscious assumptions that control their thinking, or a clinical theory, psychological concepts we use to direct and correct our clinical thinking. This folk theory problem is not unique to beginning therapists. Everyone has unconscious biases and heuristics that control their reasoning (Kahneman, 2011). Whether the subject is math, physics, or history, students must let go of misconceptions to learn concepts in their new field (Hartman, 2001). Then, they can learn to think critically in that area of expertise.

In contrast to thinking driven by unconscious folk concepts, expert clinicians use psychological concepts for clinical thinking. And they may use several different listening methods to analyze the patient's words and behaviors. They do not make things up based on assumptions. They construct hypotheses *based on evidence from the patient*. They do not treat hypotheses as facts to believe but as questions to test. When they intervene, they ask, "Did the patient's feedback confirm my hypothesis?" If it did not, they use the feedback to change their thinking and interventions. Thus, integrating the patient's responses constantly informs and changes their understanding. In this scientific form of thinking, we learn to learn from the patient (Casement, 1992; Langs, 1989a, 1989b).

A psychotherapy model is based on a psychological theory. That theory explains human development, personality, psychopathology, and its treatment. A theory includes hierarchically organized concepts that we use for clinical thinking. And listening approaches and intervention strategies flow out of those concepts.

Therapists use a theory of psychology to *conceptualize* human situations and experiences. For instance, psychodynamic therapists use concepts such as anxiety, defenses, and transference. Maladaptive cognitions, response prevention, and schema are concepts used in cognitive-behavioral therapy. Behavioral therapists use concepts such as stimulus, habit, and behavior chain analysis.

A theory of development enables therapists to understand how trauma will affect the child at the ages of two, seven, or fifteen. How will it affect her later in adulthood? How does early development influence adult relationships? A theory of personality allows us to understand what causes a personality disorder. A theory of psychopathology helps us figure out the conflicts causing the patient's symptoms. What defenses shall we address? What maladaptive relational patterns arise, and how shall we treat them? Finally, a theory of technique tells us how to translate theory into practice. How do we use clinical thinking to intervene? What interventions can we use, and for which defenses or relational problems? What listening approaches? With whom and when do we use them, and for what purpose? How do we assess whether patients have validated our hypotheses? A scientific model of psychotherapy has methods for testing clinical hypotheses. Then, a theory is testable, reliable, and valid, thus scientific.

A psychological theory is not a collection of assumptions. Its hierarchically organized set of concepts is supported and refined through scientific methods of inquiry. Falsifiable hypotheses have been tested and provisionally accepted while subject to further revision. We clearly describe the theory and its hypotheses. Then, we can test them to find empirical support or evidence of its absence (Popper, 1959/2014). Despite debates about scientific inquiry and its methods, expert clinicians agree: we cannot simply make things up (Gill, 1983a, 1983b; Hofman, Hayes, & Lorscheid, 2021; Langs, 1989a, 1989b; Raney, 1983; Rubovitz-Seitz, 2002; Smith, 2019). We test the evidence for our hypotheses to assess their validity.

Yet, learning a psychological theory is not enough. Students need help to learn how to use theory as a tool for clinical thinking. For example, let's consider a student concerned about a patient who missed sessions.

Teacher: The patient missed two sessions. Where is that on his triangle of conflict (Malan, 1979): feelings, anxiety, or defense? [*Help the student use the concept of conflict to understand the clinical fact: missing sessions.*]

Student: Defense.

Teacher: And so what is the conflict? [*Help the student use the concept of conflict to understand why the patient missed sessions.*]

Student: I don't know.

Teacher: Does the patient want to come to therapy? [*Offer a prompt.*]

Student: Yes.

Teacher: Of course. After all, he is here! So he wants to come to therapy (*the wish*). He becomes anxious. And what defense wards off his anxiety about coming? [*Help the student use the concept of conflict to understand the patient's plight.*]

Student: Missing sessions.

Teacher: Exactly. Let's see if we can develop a hypothesis for why he misses. When the session started, he talked about a psychologist he feared would judge him. Then, he described a critical boss. How might he perceive you if those two people symbolize how he feels about therapy? [*Help the student use the concepts of transference and latent content to understand the clinical fact: missing the sessions.*]

Student: Oh. He is afraid I'll judge and criticize him. [*The student can analyze latent content to see the transference.*]

Teacher: How does that change your understanding of why he misses sessions? [*Helping the student use the latent content to understand the clinical fact: missing sessions.*]

Student: I hadn't realized he was afraid I'll judge him. Now, this makes more sense.

In this example, the student learned to use concepts of conflict, transference, and latent content to see why the patient missed sessions. And once she knew the cause, she could address it. The instructor's questions taught the student how to use concepts for clinical thinking to understand and solve a psychological problem.

The learning process moves from lower to higher levels of conceptualizing, each connected to the next. First she saw the defense, then the conflict, then the unconscious transference. Finally, she saw the automatic patterns causing the patient's problems. As a result, she could intervene more effectively.

Every genuine psychotherapy model relies on a comprehensive theory of psychology. The therapist uses concepts from that theory to engage in clinical thinking. In psychodynamic therapy, lower-order concepts include feelings, anxiety, and defense. Then, the teacher teaches a higher-order concept, such as conflict. This concept enables the student to perceive a pattern: *feelings* trigger *anxiety* and *defenses*. The three lower-order concepts form a higher-order concept. Next, the teacher teaches another concept: *transference*. Now, the student perceives another pattern. The same conflict occurs in the patient's past, present, and therapy relationships. One can see a similar hierarchical structure in schema therapy (Young, Klosko, & Weishaar, 2003). Cognitions and perceptions are lower-order concepts. Schema, a higher-order concept, reveals a pattern of cognitions and perceptions across relationships.

Step One: The student learns lower-order concepts: *feelings*, *anxiety*, and *defense*.

Step Two: The student learns how the concept of *conflict* organizes feelings, anxiety, and defense into a pattern.

Step Three: The student can use the concept of *transference* to perceive a pattern of conflicts across relationships.

In cognitive/behavioral therapy:

Step One: The student learns a lower-order concept: *maladaptive thoughts*.
Step Two: The student learns how the concept of *schema* organizes thoughts and behaviors into a pattern of relatedness.
Step Three: The student learns the principle of *response prevention* to address the schema in the here and now.

The instructor teaches concepts step by step from lower to higher orders of abstraction. When students understand how those concepts function together as an interrelated system, they see how a theory works.

I will use psychodynamic theory to illustrate principles of teaching and supervision. However, these principles apply to any treatment model based on a comprehensive psychological theory, for example cognitive/behavioral therapy.

The Hierarchical Structure of Clinical Thinking and Knowledge

A comprehensive psychological theory has a hierarchically organized set of concepts that allows us to engage in levels of conceptual thinking. Let's use psychodynamic theory to illustrate the levels of conceptual thinking.

Table 2.1 Levels of conceptualization within clinical thinking

---

Clinical facts: Thoughts, feelings, and behaviors of the patient and therapist.
Lower-order concepts: *Abstract scientific concepts we use to understand clinical facts.* These concepts include stimuli, feelings, anxiety, defense, and transference.
Higher-order concepts: (*These reveal a pattern that connects lower-order concepts.*) For example:

—— Conflict reveals how feelings, anxiety, and defense form a pattern.
—— Process shows whether a statement promotes or inhibits free association.
—— Causality reveals how the sequence of stimulus, feelings, anxiety, and defenses causes presenting problems and symptoms.

Supra-ordinate concepts a: (*These meta-level concepts reveal patterns of higher-level concepts.*) For example:

—— Transference reveals a pattern of conflicts (higher-order concept) across relationships.
—— A resistance system refers to patterns of defense (higher-order concept) such as isolation of affect, repression, and splitting and projection.

(*Continued*)

Table 2.1 (Continued)

Supra-ordinate concepts b: (*These reveal patterns of supra-ordinate concepts.*) For example:

——*Level of character pathology*: therapists can understand a pattern of conflict, transference, defense, and countertransference as a neurotic, borderline, or psychotic level of character structure.

Principles of intervention: (*Principles derived from the underlying concepts that guide procedural knowledge.*) For example:

——Work from the surface to the depth. Start with what the patient sees to what she doesn't see.
——Make sure the patient wants to engage in therapy.
——Deactivate misperceptions of the therapist to develop a therapeutic alliance.
——Assess each response to an intervention to see whether it confirmed a hypothesis.

Theory: *Theory links concepts into a system of meaning-making that explains the causes of patients' symptoms. Concepts are tools we use for clinical thinking to generate hypotheses. Then, we test hypotheses through interventions to heal the patient. And as we will see, clinical thinking integrates cognitive and affective skills.*

Students learn concepts best when we teach the simplest first and the most complex last. Then students can see how a theory creates a holistic pattern of thinking and perception.

For instance, a patient says she is empty of feelings. The teacher can invite students to use simple concepts to analyze that statement.

Teacher: The patient says she is empty of feelings. Is that statement a feeling, anxiety in the body, or a defense? [*Teaching the student to use a concept (conflict) to think about a clinical fact (a patient says she is empty of feelings).*]

Student: Defense. [*The student learns to use a concept, defense, to analyze the function of the patient's statement, "I am empty of feelings."*]

Teacher: Yes. The patient can present as if she is empty of feelings. If we see her defense, what is the conflict she described? In other words, what feelings arose, where did she feel her anxiety, and what defense did she use? [*The teacher invites the student to use a more complex concept, conflict, to understand the patient further.*]

Student: When her boyfriend rejected her, that would have triggered feelings. They make her anxious and tense. So she avoids her feelings by emptying herself. [*The student develops a broader understanding.*]

Teacher: When she presents as if she is an emotionally empty woman, what kind of relationship does she invite you to have? [*The teacher invites the student to use another complex concept: transference.*]

Student: Oh. She invites me to relate to an emotionally empty person.
Teacher: And what kind of relationship would you have?
Student: An emotionally empty relationship, where she withholds from me.

Now, the student sees the transference, its function as a defense, and how it could defeat the therapy. As a result, he is more motivated to point it out and address it.

Step by step, the student learns how different concepts enrich his understanding of the patient. And he sees how these concepts form a system of clinical thinking and intervention. He begins to understand the theory's hierarchical structure.

The Process of Clinical Thinking

Psychotherapists think clinically *to diagnose the sequence of causality.* What causes the patient's presenting problems and symptoms? To answer this question, the clinician observes the patient's responses to intervention. "When I intervene, does she respond with feelings, anxiety, defenses, relational patterns, or symptoms?" Then, the therapist analyzes each response to diagnose what causes the patient's symptoms. What interventions or stimuli trigger feelings and anxiety in the session? How do anxiety and defenses create the patient's symptoms and presenting problems? What transferences are damaging the patient's intimate relationships?

Next, therapists can form a hypothesis and test it through interventions. Every intervention tests a hypothesis. Interventions allow us to discover what feelings trigger anxiety, defenses, and symptoms. Does the patient require anxiety regulation? Can the patient see the defense? Does she understand how this defense creates her symptom? Thus, interventions constitute a form of sequential experimentation. And these experiments generate an iterative learning process. Each patient response changes and refines our understanding throughout every session (Box, Hunter, & Hunter, 2005; Fisher, 1952; Simpson, 2014).

Then, *therapists analyze the patient's responses to intervention.* What did the patient's response teach me? Suppose a patient suffers from pathological grief. What defenses make her depressed right now? Does that pattern occur elsewhere in the patient's life? Clinicians look for consistent patterns in patients' words, behaviors, and relationships that cause symptoms. Then, therapists can develop a hypothesis connecting these patterns throughout the patient's life (Bateson, 2000).

Finally, the therapist assesses whether the patient's responses confirm or disconfirm hypotheses. If not, we can change our hypotheses and interventions to tune in better to the patient. As we refine our hypotheses, our understanding of the patient improves. As a result, we can be more effective. Integrating the patient's feedback helps us change our thinking and interventions. Thus, clinical thinking and metacognition (critical thinking about our thinking) are inextricably intertwined.

Based on these observed patterns, the field develops general psychological laws and theories that are broadly applicable. For instance,

When patients face what they usually avoid, anxiety rises.
Defenses can cause presenting problems and symptoms.
The less feeling a patient can bear inside, the more he will project outside.

These and other patterns allow us to define cause-effect relationships. And we refer to these forms of determination as laws. "Laws do not determine anything; *they are the forms or patterns of determination*" (Bunge, 2009, p. 23).

As research continues, clinical theory develops and changes. Skilled clinicians do not stick with one simplistic way to understand patients. When they learn something new, they revise their previous knowledge to intervene in new ways. As knowledge changes and grows, clinicians change, too (adapted from Paul & Elder, 2019). However, many factors influence whether we refine our hypotheses (Kuhn, 1962).

The Development of Expertise in Clinical Thinking

Knowledge acquisition and clinical thinking go hand in hand (Boshuizen & Schmidt, 1992, 2016; Schmidt & Boshuizen, 1993). Each theoretical concept provides practical possibilities. For example, conflict offers a new way to represent the patient's difficulties: the patient's feelings trigger anxiety, and defenses rise to ward off anxiety. But the defenses cause the patient's presenting problems. The student learns how to listen for conflict in the patient's words and deeds. And she acquires new skills to describe and analyze conflicts. However, it takes time for students to integrate concepts and the intervention skills they provide (Boshuizen & van der Wiel, 1998).

First, the student learns several concepts, listening skills, and interventions. Next, she can make connections between different concepts. When the student frequently connects these concepts and patterns, they cluster together. Now, the student can make direct links, skipping intermediate concepts.

Through this "knowledge encapsulation" (Boshuizen & Schmidt, 2016), assessments become quicker and more automatic. Now the student can link patient responses to concepts that "have the status of hypotheses or diagnoses in their reasoning process" (Boshuizen & Schmidt, 2016, p. 59). The student no longer laboriously works through each step in clinical thinking.

Instead, she begins to see larger patterns—scripts that allow automatic processing. However, these scripts require constant attention.

"Clinical reasoning ... is thus affected by the features of the case and the validity and structure of the knowledge base" (Boshuizen & Schmidt, 2016). And to learn this, the student requires an expert (Mayer, 2004). Teachers help students develop adequate knowledge structures (Boshuizen & Schmidt, 2016) by asking several questions. What does the student know? What does she not know? How is her knowledge structured? What is the most important piece of knowledge she could learn today?

A mix of practical experience and theoretical education is necessary (Boshuizen & Schmidt, 1992). Students learn to think clinically about patients by using concepts to collect and analyze information in cases. This clinical thinking allows them to diagnose the causes of symptoms and develop a treatment plan. Next, they intervene and analyze the patient's responses to interventions to improve their hypotheses.

Why Critical Thinking Is Rare

Critical thinking is rare in most fields (Paul & Elder, 2019). So, what factors interfere with it in the field of psychotherapy? First, a dominant theoretical framework unifies many disciplines. Second, gatekeepers reject works not conforming to that framework, thus securing the field's boundaries. For example, physicists agree upon and use the theory of quantum mechanics. However, psychotherapists do not agree upon or use a shared theory. In fact, some therapy approaches do not even have a theory.

Without a shared theory to create a boundary or gatekeepers to enforce it, the boundaries for this field are porous and fragmented. As a result, it cannot prevent invasions by ideas from other disciplines. (See Bender & Schorsk, 1997, for an analysis of knowledge domains and their boundaries.) To differentiate influence from invasion, consider the following. Studying the work of the theologian Paul Tillich deepens our understanding of dialogue. Other fields influence us. However, some practitioners rely upon prayer rather than clinical thinking. They engage in spiritual direction based on theology, not psychotherapy based on psychology. Without a unifying theory for the field, practitioners may practice without a theory to guide their clinical thinking.

A psychotherapy model is based on a theory of development, personality, and technique. However, collections of techniques without a comprehensive psychological theory often substitute for *therapy models*. Then, students lack the tools for clinical thinking that could guide their interventions. As a result, psychotherapy devolves into applying a technique to an object. And if there are only one or two techniques, no thinking is necessary about which strategy to use or why.

For instance, focusing (Gendlin, 1998) is a technique—reflection. Gendlin's texts are among the best on reflection. However, is an intervention (reflection) a model of psychotherapy? Can one intervention be sufficient for all clinical problems? Can one listening approach substitute for a theory of technique?

Gendlin bases his approach on the work of Martin Heidegger (Kleinberg-Levin, 1997). But is a philosophical theory of language a psychological theory of human functioning? Without a comprehensive theory of psychology, where do we find the concepts used for clinical thinking?

Or we could consider neuro-linguistic programming. This pseudo-scientific approach has no theory of development, causation, technique, or assessment. It uses outdated metaphors for brain functioning that are inconsistent with neuroscience. Its hypotheses are unproven, speculative ideas unsupported by research (Lilienfeld et al., 2012; Thyer, Pignotti, & Monica, 2015). It is a collection of techniques masquerading as a model of therapy.

Polyvagal theory (Porges, 2011) enriches our understanding of anxiety. But is a theory about anxiety a comprehensive theory of psychotherapy? Is a theory of the central nervous system a theory of technique? Anxiety is an essential part of any psychological theory of human functioning, but can a part substitute for the whole?

Thus, a teacher tasked with teaching an approach can ask herself several questions. Does this model have a theory with psychological concepts for clinical thinking? Does it have a theory of child development to explain the origins of psychological conditions? Is there a theory of technique flexible enough to address a wide range of psychopathology? Does this approach use multiple intervention strategies targeted to different patient capacities? Does the model include multiple listening strategies? Does it possess a theory for assessing whether patients' responses confirm or disconfirm hypotheses? Does it have a theory to analyze therapist behaviors contributing to treatment failure or dropout? Is there a method for using patient feedback to change one's thinking and hypotheses? If so, you are teaching a psychotherapy model based on a comprehensive theory of psychology.

With over 400 types of therapy, we lack the space to continue this analysis. However, many therapy brands lack a psychological theory to guide their interventions. According to some brands, one can just pray, tap fingers on a meridian, or repeat the patient's last words. Of course, students can learn such techniques from a book or a weekend conference. But we would never consider a single skill enough for any other profession as complex as psychotherapy.

When techniques lack a theory, it seems irrelevant, leading to no practical action. So, expert teachers show students how to use psychological concepts for clinical thinking to create effective interventions. When clinical concepts allow us to understand the patient more deeply, interventions become ways we relate to people to form a healing relationship.

Summary

Clinical thinking has a purpose: to find and treat the causes of psychological problems. Thus, we teach students how to use theory and concepts (declarative knowledge) for clinical thinking. Next, we teach them how to translate clinical thinking into interventions (procedural knowledge) and when and why to intervene (conditional knowledge). Finally, we teach students how to evaluate their thinking and interventions (metacognitive knowledge).

Clinical thinking in psychotherapy has a specific form due to its area of focus, knowledge, language, and theory. Further, due to its emphases, psychotherapy has unique skills and rules for seeking and testing knowledge (Davison, Pray, & Bristol, 1990; Donald, 2002; Gill, 1983a, 1983b; Gray, 1994; Jones, 2015; Langs, 1989a, 1989b; McPeck, 1981; Moore, 2015; Raney, 1983; Smith, 2018).

Some might imagine that clinical thinking does not require a theory. But even laypersons rely on preconceptions and assumptions to think about people. Those who dislike or claim to get by without a theory are in the grip of an older one. When therapists say they don't need a theory, they aren't aware of the implicit one they believe and use (Moore, 2015).

On the one hand, the definition of *clinical thinking* is simple: the reasoning and decision-making processes associated with clinical practice (Higgs & Jensen, 2016). On the other hand, clinical thinking is complex. It involves multiple levels of conceptual thinking and many listening and intervention skills. And the therapist also develops non-cognitive emotional capacities. For instance, she learns to observe and analyze her feelings, reactions, and countertransference. Thus, clinical thinking is simple and complex (Higgs, 2006).

For students to learn to use a psychological theory for clinical thinking, first, we help them become aware of the implicit, unscientific ideas they believe. By unlearning misconceptions, they can learn psychological concepts. Then, clinical thinking rather than unconscious habit can guide their interventions.

References

Bateson, G. (2000). *Steps to an ecology of mind: Collected essays in anthropology, psychiatry, evolution, and epistemology.* Chicago: University of Chicago Press.
Bender, T. & Schorsk, C. (Eds.). (1997). *American academic culture in transformation: Fifty years, four disciplines.* Princeton, N.J.: Princeton University Press.

Boshuizen, H., & Schmidt, H. (1992). On the role of biomedical knowledge in the clinical reasoning of experts, intermediates, and novices. *Cognitive Science, 16,* 153–184.

Boshuizen, H., & Schmidt, H. (2016). The development of clinical reasoning expertise. In J. Higgs, G. Jensen, S. Loftus, & N. Christensen (Eds.), *Clinical reasoning in the health professions* (4th ed., pp. 57–65). Edinburgh: Elsevier.

Boshuizen, H., & van der Wiel, M. (1998). Multiple representations in medicine: How students struggle with it. In M. van Sommeren, P. Reimann, H. Boshuizen, & T. De Jong (Eds.), *Learning with multiple representations* (pp. 237–262). Amsterdam: Elsevier.

Box, G., Hunter, J., & Hunter, W. (2005). *Statistics for experimenters* (2nd ed.). Hoboken, N.J.: Wiley and Sons.

Bunge, M. (2009). *Causality and modern science* (4th ed.). New Brunswick, N.J.: Transaction Publishers.

Casement, P. (1992). *Learning from the patient.* New York: Guilford Press.

Davison, W. T., Bristol, C., & Pray, M. (1986). Turning aggression on the self: A study of psychoanalytic process. *The Psychoanalytic Quarterly, 55*(2), 273–295.

Davison, W. T., Pray, M., & Bristol, C. (1990). Mutative interpretation and close process monitoring in a study of psychoanalytic process. *The Psychoanalytic Quarterly, 59*(4), 599–628.

DiTomaso, N. (1982). "Sociological reductionism" from Parsons to Althusser: Linking action and structure in social theory. *American Sociological Review, 47*(1), 14–28.

Donald, J. (2002). *Learning to think: Disciplinary perspectives.* San Francisco: Jossey Bass.

Engel, G. (1980). The clinical application of the biopsychosocial model. *American Journal of Psychiatry, 137,* 135–144.

Facione, P. (1990). Critical thinking: A statement of expert consensus for purposes of educational assessment and instruction. American Philosophical Association, Delphi Report. chrome-extension://efaidnbmnnnibpcajpcglclefindmkaj/ https://www.qcc.cuny.edu/socialSciences/ppecorino/CT-Expert-Report.pdf

Facione, N., & Facione, P. (2008). *Critical thinking and clinical reasoning in the health sciences: An international multidisciplinary teaching anthology.* Millbrae, Calif.: California Academic Press.

Fisher, R. (1952). Sequential experimentation. *Biometrics, 8,* 183–187.

Freud, A. (1936). *The ego and the mechanisms of defense.* New York: Norton.

Gendlin, E. (1998). *Focusing-oriented psychotherapy: A manual of the experiential method.* New York: Guilford Press.

Gill, M. & Hoffman, I. (1983a). *Analysis of transference, Vol. 1.* New York: International Universities Press.

Gill, M. & Hoffman, I. (1983b). *Analysis of transference, Vol. 2.* New York: International Universities Press.

Gray, P. (1994). *The ego and the analysis of defense.* New York: Aronson.

Hartman, H. (2001). Teaching metacognitively. In H. Hartman (Ed.), *Metacognition in learning and instruction: Theory, research, and practice* (pp. 149–169). Dordrecht, Netherlands: Kluwer Academic Publishers.

Hawkins, D., Elder, L., & Paul, R. (2010). *The thinker's guide to clinical reasoning.* Dillon, Calif.: The Foundation for Critical Thinking.

Hayes, N. (1995). Reductionism in psychological theory. In N. Hayes (Ed.), *Psychology in perspective* (pp. 1–18). London: Red Globe Press.

Higgs, J. (2006). The complexity of clinical reasoning: Exploring the dimensions of clinical reasoning expertise as a situated, lived phenomenon. Seminar presented at the Faculty of Health Sciences, University of Sidney, Australia, May 5.

Higgs, J., & Jensen, G. (2016). Clinical reasoning: Challenges of interpretation and practice in the 21st century. In J. Higgs, G. Jensen, S. Loftus, & N. Christensen (Eds.), *Clinical reasoning in the health professions* (4th ed., pp. 3–12). Edinburgh: Elsevier.

Hofman, S., Hayes, S., & Lorscheid, D. (2021). *Learning process-based therapy: A skills training manual for targeting the core processes of psychological change in clinical practice.* Oakland, Calif.: Context Press.

Jones, A. (2015). A disciplined approach to critical thinking. In M. Davies & R. Barnett (Eds.), *The Palgrave handbook of critical thinking in higher education* (pp. 169–182). New York: Palgrave MacMillan.

Kahneman, D. (2011). *Thinking, fast and slow.* New York: Farrar, Straus, and Giroux.

Kleinberg-Levin, D. (Ed.). (1997). *Language beyond postmodernism: Saying and thinking in Gendlin's philosophy.* Evanston, Ill.: Northwestern University Press.

Kuhn, T. (1962). *The structure of scientific revolutions.* Chicago: University of Chicago Press.

Langs, R. (1989a). *The technique of psychoanalytic psychotherapy: Vol. 1. Initial contact: Theoretical framework: Understanding the patient's communications: The therapist's interventions.* New York: Aronson.

Langs, R. (1989b). *The technique of psychoanalytic psychotherapy: Vol. 2. Responses to interventions: Patient-therapist relationship: Phases of psychotherapy.* New York: Aronson.

Levenson, E. (1972). *The fallacy of understanding.* New York: Basic Books.

Levenson, E. (1984). *The ambiguity of change: An inquiry into the nature of psychoanalytic reality.* New York: Basic Books.

Levenson, E. (1991). *The purloined self: Interpersonal perspective in psychoanalysis.* New York: Basic Books.

Lilienfeld, S., Ammirati, R., & David, M. (2012). Distinguishing science from pseudo-science in school psychology: Science and scientific thinking as safeguards against human error. *Journal of School Psychology, 1,* 7–36.

Loewald, H. (1989). *Papers on psychoanalysis.* New Haven, Conn.: Yale University Press.

Malan, D. (1979). *Individual psychotherapy and the science of psychodynamics* (2nd ed.). London: Butterworth-Heineman.

Mayer, R. (2004). Should there be a three-strikes rule against pure discovery learning? The case for guided methods of instruction. *American Psychologist, 59*(1), 14–19. https://doi.org/10.1037/0003-066X.59.1.14. PMID 14736316.

McPeck, J. (1981). *Critical thinking and education.* New York: St. Martin's Press.

Moore, T. (2015). Disciplinarity and the teaching of critical thinking. In R. Wegeriff & J. Kaufman (Eds.), *The Routledge international handbook of research on teaching thinking* (pp. 243–253). New York: Routledge.

Paul, R., & Elder, L. (2019). *The miniature guide to thinking concepts and tools.* Tomales, Calif.: Foundation for Critical Thinking Press.

Plato. (2005). *Phaedrus*. Trans. C. Rowe. New York: Penguin.

Popper, K. (1959/2014). *The logic of scientific discovery*. New York: Martino Fine Books.

Porges, S. (2011). *The polyvagal theory: Neurophysiological foundations of emotions, attachment, communication, and self-regulation*. New York: Norton.

Raney, J. (1983). *Listening and interpreting: The challenge of the work of Robert Langs*. New York: Aronson.

Rose, S. (1998). What is wrong with reductionist explanations of behavior? *Novartis Found Symp., 213*, 176–186.

Rubovitz-Seitz, P. (2002). *A primer of clinical interpretation: Classic and post-classic approaches*. New York: Jason Aronson.

Schmidt, H., & Boshuizen, H. (1993). On acquiring expertise in medicine. *Educational Psychology Review, 5*, 205–221.

Simpson, J. (2014). *Testing via sequential experiments: Best practice and tutorial*. Wright-Patterson AFB, Ohio: Scientific Tests and Analysis Techniques Center of Excellence.

Smith, D. (2019). *Hidden conversations: An introduction to communicative psychoanalysis*. New York: Routledge.

Thyer, B., Pignotti, A., & Monica, G. (2015). *Science and pseudoscience in social work practice*. New York: Springer.

Young, J., Klosko, J., & Weishaar, M. (2003). *Schema therapy: A practitioner's guide*. New York: Guilford.

Chapter 3

Learning Clinical Thinking by Unlearning Biases and Assumptions

Jon Frederickson

In all fields, students enter with preconceptions (Marsh & Eliseev, 2019) that conflict with the material to be learned (Goldwater & Schalk, 2016). And in medicine, cognitive biases often lead to mistakes in clinical thinking (Saposnik et al., 2016). This shift from biases is not peculiar to psychotherapy. Students must shift from misconceptions to scientific concepts in many fields (Zohar & Dori, 2012). Thus, teachers help students see and experience the limitations of their biases. Once students let go of unconscious assumptions, they can consciously use psychological concepts.

For instance, students may come to supervision wanting a technique to apply to an object. But to form a healing relationship, they need to understand the patient. So, we start with their wish for an answer. If we can show how clinical thought leads to effective action, they will want to learn how to do it.

A student complains, "I don't understand why you ask me questions. Just tell me what to do!" The student's question is the best expression of his learning need. Start there.

Student: What should I say to my patient?

Teacher: That's the right question to ask. [*Validate the wish to learn, no matter what form it takes.*] Let's see what is going on in order to figure out what to say. [*Then pivot to the educational task.*] You asked what the patient wanted help with. And she said she had a list of things to work on, but she had forgotten them. When she said she had forgotten her problem, was that the problem? Or is it a defense against declaring a problem? [*Questions teach the student how to think clinically about patient responses.*]

Student: A defense.

Teacher: If she forgets her problem, can she work on it? [*A question teaches the student to see the price of the patient's defense.*]

Student: We couldn't work on a problem if she didn't describe one.

Teacher: How might you say that to her? [*Inviting the student to design an intervention based on the clinical thinking he did.*]

DOI: 10.4324/9781003488637-3

Student: If you don't know what the problem is, we won't be able to work on one.

Teacher: How could you invite her again to share her problem?

Student: What problem would you like me to help you with?

Teacher: What did you learn about how to deal with the patient's defense against declaring a problem? [*Inviting the student to think about his learning (metacognition). How does this new information change his old knowledge?*]

Student: I need to show her the price of the defense and then ask the question again.

Teacher: How does this change your understanding of how to address defenses against declaring a problem? [*Inviting the student to think about the change in his knowledge (metacognition). He has integrated his learning at a higher level. Can he understand a technique within an over-arching principle?*]

Student: I was stuck and thought maybe I had to wait until she declared a problem. [*His layperson assumption: "There is no conflict, so if I wait, the patient will tell the problem."*] But you're saying I can point out the price of the defense and ask for the problem again. [*He sees the technique but has not integrated it within the principle. Also, we do not know if his folk assumption has resolved.*]

Teacher: And what impact would your intervention have on the therapeutic focus?

Student: Oh, right. If I keep returning to the problem, we won't wander all over the place. [*He understands the principle guiding the intervention: maintain a therapeutic focus.*]

Teacher: And why didn't waiting work? [*Has his assumption changed?*]

Student: She used defenses.

Teacher: So instead of waiting, you can ...

Student: Point out the defenses. [*His assumption has changed. So, his work should change.*]

The expert clinician's interventions may seem purely intuitive. However, they result from an implicit process of assessment that has become automatized. Thus, the expert teacher reverse engineers this process. Then, she can teach students the steps of clinical thinking through decision tree questions.

Table 3.1 Example of decision tree questions in the previous example

Clinical thinking question: When she said she had forgotten her problem, was that the problem? Or is it a defense against declaring a problem?
Clinical thinking question: If she forgets her problem, can she work on it?
Intervention prompt: How might you point out that if she forgets a problem, we wouldn't have one to work on, and then invite her to share a problem?

Decision tree questions illustrate the sequence of questions an expert asks to diagnose the patient's psychological problems. By asking these questions step by step, the instructor teaches the steps of clinical thinking. Decision tree questions (Lemov, 2021) invite students to use concepts to engage in clinical thinking. In this form of instruction, we don't teach the answers. Instead, we teach the questions by which we generate hypotheses. Decision tree questions make students think aloud, learning each step in clinical thinking.

In this case, the student learned to use the concept of conflict to analyze a patient's statement. Then, he saw the price of the defense. As a result, he knows how to point out the price of the defense and invite the patient to declare a problem. His clinical thinking has led to an effective intervention.

Decision tree questions: The sequence of questions an expert asks when doing clinical thinking. The expert uses these questions to assess the patient's responses. This analysis informs her next intervention.

Decision tree questions as teaching device: The sequence of questions teaches students the steps in clinical thinking. Any question students cannot answer tells the teacher the step in clinical thinking where they need help. Thus, the questions function as both a teaching and an assessment tool.

Teachers may judge students for their seeming concreteness. For instance, it would be easy to assume the student's concreteness is a problem about learning (Ekstein & Wallerstein, 1972), an emotional attitude blocking his learning. Yet, if we think about his thinking, we can identify his learning problem (Ekstein & Wallerstein, 1972), the most basic skill or concept he could learn today. Or we can find the folk assumption or bias creating that seeming concreteness. The previous student could not use the concept of conflict to analyze the patient's responses. As a result, he could not see the defense and return to the therapeutic focus. Thus, the decision tree questions focused on that skill.

In addition, his preconceptions kept the therapy stuck. He thought if he waited, the patient would declare a problem. He assumed that conscious will was enough. He also assumed that no unconscious factors interfered with the patient's will. He also assumed that his waiting strategy would work while ignoring the evidence that it didn't. Thus, he assumed that he did not have to assess the patient's responses to his interventions. This example illustrates how one misconception often connects to others.

The student did not know that defenses could prevent the patient from declaring a problem. And he did not realize he could block defenses to help the patient declare a problem. Once his preconception (waiting) was corrected and replaced by the concepts of conflict and defense work, he could help the patient.

Unlearning folk concepts requires students to challenge their assumptions, question previous beliefs, and let go of habits that prevent them from being effective therapists. That process is always difficult because unlearning challenges a way of thinking, listening, and relating that has been adaptive for at least twenty-five years. Unexamined assumptions, habits, and biases provide a false certainty about complex issues. In this case, the situation appeared simple to the student. He thought he should wait. He did not see the complexity: the patient wanted to share a problem, and defenses prevented her from doing so. His unconscious assumption determined what he could perceive, think, and understand. When we help students see and let go of their unconscious assumptions and habits, they can consciously use psychological concepts for clinical thinking.

Folk Concepts versus Scientific Concepts

Every culture has an implicit "folk" psychology (Churchland, 1998; Fletcher, 1995) composed of assumptions that allow us to understand other people. These notions seem like common sense to the beginning student: natural, obvious, and universal. Yet those beliefs are natural only in the specific historical, cultural, and social context of the student's background (Lundholm, 2018).

Students enter psychotherapy training with unconscious assumptions and biases that direct their non-scientific thinking. These implicit narratives are widely accepted in the student's background. To her, her thoughts are just how things are. She may not realize that preconceptions guide her thinking.

Some refer to laypersons' preconceptions as a folk psychology (Churchland, 1998; Fletcher, 1995). However, others suggest that these misconceptions do not form a coherent whole (Kottler and Balkin, 2020). Instead, laypersons' ideas consist of many quasi-independent elements (Hartman, 2001; diSessa, 2022). Why is this important? The student may equate folk concepts with clinical concepts.

Therefore, the teacher engages in critical thinking. What folk concepts does the student use? Is she aware of those concepts? How do they influence her thinking? Does she treat her thought as a belief or as a hypothesis to test? However, teachers may miss certain biases because the layperson uses well-known words like feelings, anxiety, and listening, which are folk concepts with a general, popularly understood meaning.

Clinical concepts have a formal and specific definition within the theory of psychology. And they have been refined through research. They almost always differ from the folk concepts students already know. For instance, the layman's use of the term "feeling" is broad and vague. However, the clinical concept of "feeling" is quite limited and specific, understood within a psychological theory based on research. Thus, it has great depth and complexity (e.g., Damasio, 2000; Ekman, 2003; Kernberg, 2001; Solms, 2021).

The layman's folk concept of anxiety consists of worries and thoughts. In psychodynamic theory, however, anxiety is not a thought but a feeling. Moreover, anxiety has a specific function. It signals that dangerous unconscious feelings, impulses, or thoughts are rising to awareness (S. Freud, 1923/1961a, 1926/1961b; A. Freud, 1936). Further, we understand it as an unconscious (Damasio, 2000; LeDoux, 1998) bio-physiological discharge pattern in the body mediated by the somatic and autonomic nervous systems (Abbass, 2015; Habib Davanloo, personal supervision 2002–2004; Frederickson, 2013, 2020; Janig, 2008; Porges, 2011; Robertson et al., 2004). (Of course, other therapy models may describe this concept differently. See Barlow & Fanchione [2017].)

Likewise, the folk concept of listening differs from clinical listening in psychotherapy. Suppose a layperson hears a patient ask, "What should I do?" The layperson listens to the *manifest content*. He hears the conscious meaning—a simple request for advice that means nothing else.

However, the expert clinician listens from multiple perspectives to assess the unconscious context in which a conscious request occurs (Frederickson, 1999; Langs, 1989a, 1989b; Matte Blanco, 1975; Paniagua, 1991; Tansey & Burke, 1995). For example, suppose the patient spoke freely about his ambition to attend art school. Then he shifted and asked his therapist, "What should I do?"

The beginning student, listening only to the manifest content, might answer the question and encourage the patient to go to art school. However, the expert clinician engages in *clinical* listening from several perspectives. As a result, she can assess conscious *and* unconscious meanings and processes. Multiple listening skills can help students tailor their listening approach to the patient's unique needs. Here are other listening perspectives the expert clinician may use.

Listening to the process. Here, we listen to the sequence of associations to assess the *function* of that sentence, "What should I do?" Did his question help him express his opinion about art school? Or did he invite the therapist to offer hers? The question may have had an inhibiting *function*. It may have inhibited the patient's freedom to describe his desire (A. Freud, 1936; Davison, Bristol, & Pray, 1986; Davison, Pray, & Bristol, 1990; Gray, 1994). The clinician could test this hypothesis. "You are asking for my opinion now, but a moment ago, you were freer to discuss your own.

I wonder if something felt risky about revealing your opinion about art school here with me?"

Listening to the conflict. From this perspective, we listen to the wish, fear, and defense depicted in the manifest content. Suppose the patient says his parents object to his ambition. The therapist might form a hypothesis. The patient wants to go to art school. He fears his parents' disapproval. So, as a defense, he questions his desire like his parents do.

Listening to the latent content. Here, we listen to see if the patient's words symbolize his unconscious experience of therapy. For example, he describes his ambition. But he may fear that the therapist (like his parents) would oppose his desires. Thus, he inhibits himself in the therapist's presence.

Listening to the enactment: Suppose the patient tends to take a one-down position with people. The therapist might wonder if the patient's question enacts a one-down role in therapy. So, the therapist would not give advice since it might invite the patient to take a one-down role (Havens, 1986). And we would not find out what makes the patient anxious about owning his authority. Here, we listen to the patient's words and the enactment they invite.

Listening to the countertransference: Here, the clinician listens to her feelings and thoughts. Do they symbolize the patient's conflict or hers? For example, suppose she noticed an urge to tell the patient what to do. She might wonder, "Why do *I* feel such a strong urge to offer my opinion when this is *his* problem? Why does *his* conflict feel so dangerous that I want to make it disappear? Why am I tempted to act like his parents and tell him what to do?" (Ogden, 1992; Racker, 1968).

Beginning therapists who listen to the manifest content often assume that words have only a literal meaning. And that assumption determines what they can hear and think about.

As therapists learn additional listening skills, they develop more perspectives on the patient's problems (Frederickson, 1999; Paniagua, 1991). As a result, their thinking and understanding become more flexible. They begin to see the unconscious context in which a conscious question arises (Frederickson, 1999; Paniagua, 1991; Tansey & Burke, 1995). A folk concept of listening for a conscious, literal meaning shifts to a clinical concept of *also* listening for unconscious, symbolic meanings.

This example illustrates how folk concepts and psychological concepts differ. The layperson habitually listens to manifest content. The expert clinician consciously listens from multiple perspectives. The layperson treats his opinion as a truth to believe. The clinician treats an opinion as a *hypothesis* to test. The layperson treats words as if they have only a conscious literal meaning. The expert clinician listens to both conscious and unconscious meanings in the patient's words and behaviors.

The student operates according to a folk belief: answer a question. The expert operates according to a *principle*: analyze the psychological context in which the question occurs. We adhere neither to the dogmatic belief that one should answer a question nor the conviction that one should not. Instead, we use multiple listening perspectives to assess the *psychological context* for a question. Rather than dogma determining our reaction, clinical thought can inform our response.

The beginning student does not know the differences between a folk concept of listening and a clinical concept. Thus, teaching the differences between folk and clinical concepts is essential. Then, the student can learn the unique skills of clinical listening.

The student's preconceptions differ from the explicit concepts in many disciplines (Hartman, 2001; Hiebert & Lefevre, 1986; Kottler & Balkin, 2020). Therefore, clinical concepts often feel counterintuitive. For instance, a student listened passively while the patient avoided declaring a problem to work on. The teacher suggested she might address those defenses. However, the student thought this would be insensitive. The teacher realized the student needed help differentiating between folk and

Table 3.2 Listening perspectives used in clinical listening

Listening Perspectives	Definitions
Listening to manifest content	Listening to the patient's words literally without any extra meanings implied.
Listening for conflict (within the manifest content)	Listening to content to see if the patient's words depict a conflict between feelings/desires, anxiety, and defense.
Listening for process	Listening to the sequence of the patient's associations. The therapist examines the function of a patient's statement. Does it express his desire or inhibit it (*defense*)?
Listening for latent content	Listening to see if the patient's words symbolize his experience of the therapist. The patient describes his parents' disapproval of his ambition. Thus, the patient may fear the therapist's disapproval, too.
Listening for enactment	Listening to see if the therapist and patient are enacting a past relationship. A therapist who reassures the patient about his ambition might enact the role of the superior/judging parent.
Listening to the countertransference	Listening to the therapist's feelings to see if they symbolize part of the patient's conflict. Suppose the therapist feels the urge to comment on the patient's desire. Rather than act on it, the therapist can wonder why she feels that urge and analyze the function it serves.

clinical concepts of sensitivity. Once she sees those assumptions and their limitations, she can learn psychological concepts to engage in clinical thinking.

Student: I think it's important to be sensitive. [*A folk concept substitutes for a clinical concept.*]

Teacher: I'm glad we agree. Shall we do a role-play so you can show us how to do that? [*Create a situation where the student can experience the effects of her bias. That experience can help her realize what to learn and why.*]

Student: Sure.

Teacher: How about I play the patient, and you play my therapist?

Student: Okay. What problem would you like me to help you with?

Teacher as the patient: My wife thinks I should be here.

Student: That must be tough.

Teacher as the patient: It is. Let's talk about her. [*Enact the problem with the student's folk concept.*]

Student: [*Puzzled.*] Could you tell me more about what your wife thinks?

Teacher as the patient: Absolutely. I would much prefer to talk about my wife instead of myself. [*Enact the problem so the student experiences it.*]

Student: I'm a bit stuck now. [*She is beginning to see how the folk concept is getting her into trouble.*]

Teacher as the patient: How so? [*Inviting her to think about her assumption.*]

Student: We seem to be getting stuck. [*The student is experiencing a problem: her strategy did not work. As a result, a learning need emerges.*]

Teacher as the patient: As your patient, what am I doing that keeps me stuck? [*Inviting her to analyze the patient's statements. Then she will understand the symptom: being stuck.*]

Student: You talked about your wife.

Teacher as the patient: When I said my wife wanted me to come, was that the problem I needed help with? Or was it a way to avoid declaring my problem? [*Inviting her to think about patient statements using the concept of conflict.*]

Student: A way to avoid.

Teacher as the patient:	Would that be the problem or a defense against declaring a problem I want to work on? [*Inviting her to think about patient statements using the concept of conflict.*]
Student:	Defense.
Teacher as the patient:	And were you sensitive to my problem or my defense? [*Inviting her to think about sensitivity from the perspective of conflict.*]
Student:	[*Pause.*] The defense.
Teacher:	If we return to the patient, he is in conflict. Insofar as he comes, he wants help with a problem. We could assume this makes him anxious. And then, he uses defenses to avoid declaring a problem. Shall we be sensitive only to his defense? Or shall we also be sensitive to his problem (the wish to get well) and his anxiety? [*Inviting her to use the concept of conflict to reflect on her folk concept.*]
Student:	Well, I definitely want to be sensitive to his wish to get well and his anxiety.
Teacher:	Of course, we want to be sensitive to his entire conflict (the wish to get well, his anxiety about that wish, and his defenses). How does this idea of conflict change your idea of being sensitive as a therapist? [*Inviting metacognition: how does new information change her old knowledge? How is her folk concept of sensitivity evolving into a psychological concept?*]
Student:	It's weird. I hadn't thought of it this way before. [*When a student uses a folk concept automatically, thinking about it is unnecessary.*]
Teacher:	As you think about it, how does this change your understanding of being a sensitive therapist? [*Inviting metacognition: how does new information change her old knowledge? How is her folk concept evolving into a psychological concept?*]
Student:	I have to be sensitive to his wish to get well, his anxiety, and his defenses. [*Now she understands sensitivity within the concept of conflict.*]
Teacher:	What will happen if you are sensitive only to his defenses?
Student:	I guess he will keep using them, and then we wouldn't learn what his problem is. [*She sees the link between her interventions and causality.*]

Teacher:	Right. Defenses would keep the two of you stuck. And if you are sensitive only to the defenses, would that be sensitive to his wish to get well? [*Inviting metacognition about her folk concept.*]
Student:	No.
Teacher:	How might you acknowledge his defense of talking about his wife's opinion and be sensitive to his wish to get help? [*Inviting her to use a psychotherapeutic concept of sensitivity to guide her interventions.*]
Student:	That's what your wife thought. But what is the problem *you* would like my help with?
Teacher:	Exactly. So, how does the concept of conflict help us be even more sensitive as therapists? [*Inviting metacognition: how does her new understanding change her folk concept of sensitivity? What has she integrated and not integrated?*]

I could have told her to block the defense and return to the therapeutic focus. But her folk concept of sensitivity would have continued to drive her reactions. Instead, when her strategy did not work in the role-play, she experienced the limitations of her approach. Thus, she wanted to learn something new. And she began to see how the concept of conflict could make her even more sensitive. Once she could empathize with the patient's wish, anxiety, and defense (A. Freud, 1936), she experienced complex empathy (Havens, 1986). I agreed with part of her folk concept of sensitivity so that we could develop it into a more complex psychological concept.

> *Principle*: Always align with the student's cherished values. Then, help her see how her folk concept conflicts with her values.

Do not get into conflict with your student's values. Instead, let her experience how her everyday thinking habits conflict with her values. When she sees how clinical thinking can help her embody her values more deeply, she will want to learn more.

Clinical thinking does not come naturally to students. Instead, they use an unscientific thinking style based on folk concepts and biases. Yet, inaccurate prior information is resistant to teaching in every field (Taylor & Kowalski, 2014). Unless instructors systematically help students integrate new information, old misconceptions remain intact. Telling students that the "correct view" leads to as little as a 5% change in students (Gutman, 1979). Folk concepts prevent students from learning new concepts. For instance, in the video, "A Private Universe," Harvard graduates believed that seasons change in response to the earth's closeness to the sun. After years of instruction, they still held onto that folk concept, never having integrated the scientific concept of the earth's tilted axis. (Video link: https://www.youtube.com/watch?v=JXb7Oq13pjQ.)

Clearly, unlearning folk concepts is harder than learning new concepts. To address that problem, we examine the preconceptions influencing students' thinking and perception. Next, we can use those assumptions in role-plays, so that a student experiences the limitations of a bias. Now, she can think about it consciously rather than use it unconsciously. And she can change her preconceptions by thinking about and analyzing them. Once she lets go of folk concepts, psychological concepts and skills can guide her clinical thinking.

Students cannot integrate new information unless old biases dissolve. When folk concepts continue to drive their therapy, students' unscientific thinking will remain unchanged, and their effectiveness will not improve. (See Taylor & Kowalski [2014] on preconceptions as obstacles to learning.)

For instance, a student mistakenly believed that describing the patient's defenses was "aggressive." As a result of this misconception, she listened to the patient's self-attacks in the session, allowing her depression to deepen.

Student: It seems aggressive to point out the patient's defenses. [*Misconception preventing the therapist from maintaining an effective therapeutic focus.*]

Teacher: That's a good point since we don't want to be aggressive in any way that would harm the patient. [*Joining with the student's values.*] As we look at this patient's situation, are you causing her depression? Or are defenses causing her depression? [*Helping the student see causality.*]

Student: Defenses?

Teacher: Right. Are you aggressive to the patient? Or are the self-attacks aggressive to the patient? [*Helping the student see the location of aggression.*]

Student: I hadn't thought of it that way. [*In unscientific thinking, we cannot think about how biases shape our thinking because they are unconscious. Or if they are conscious, they are regarded as truths to believe, not hypotheses to question.*]

Teacher: If we think of it that way, does the patient see these defenses attacking her? [*Helping the student see that defenses occur outside the patient's awareness.*]

Student: No. She's not aware of the self-attacks.

Teacher: So would you be willing to protect her from those aggressive attackers by identifying them so she could see them? [*Helping the student understand the principle behind defense work.*]

Student: When you put it that way, it makes sense.

Teacher: Sure. Imagine she was blindfolded and handcuffed, and a criminal was hitting her. Would you be willing to defend her from an attacker she couldn't see? [*Using a metaphor to help the therapist understand the therapeutic stance.*]

Student: Of course!

Teacher: And would she accuse you of being aggressive for protecting her from that criminal?

Student: [Laughs.] No.

Teacher: How does this change your understanding of defense work? [*Metacognitive question to assess what the student has integrated. Has his misconception about aggression and defense work changed?*]

Decision tree questions helped the student see that the therapist is not aggressive to the patient; defenses are. Then, she understood her therapeutic role. Defense work protects the patient from aggressive defenses. The therapist is not an aggressor but a protector.

Another student, due to a folk concept, wondered why we would address defenses to help a patient maintain an effective therapeutic focus.

Student: Don't we need to allow space for the patient to talk? [*A folk concept that is vague and general. The student does not know how to analyze the function of each patient statement: does this statement give or take space away from the patient?*]

Teacher: Absolutely! When you asked the patient about her feelings toward her abusive husband, was she able to talk about her feelings, or did thoughts come in instead? [*Can he begin to see the function of defenses?*]

Student: She talked about her thoughts.

Teacher: And when thoughts came in, did they make space for her feelings, or did they take up the space instead? [*Can he shift from thinking about space as a static folk concept to space as a dynamic psychological concept?*]

Student: But shouldn't we make space for those thoughts, too? [*He does not see the function of those thoughts: to ward off feelings. Therefore, he does not understand his therapeutic role.*]

Teacher: Good question. If we let thoughts take up the space, who will make space for her feelings? [*In a folk concept, space naturally occurs if the patient talks. Therefore, he could not see how defenses take space from the patient. As a result, he did not see what his therapeutic role would be.*]

Student: Me? [*The student is still unsure.*]

Teacher: If we let thoughts take up the space instead of feelings, what would we treat as more deserving of space: her thoughts or feelings? [*Can he see his role in the co-creation of space in therapy?*]

Student: Her thoughts. I see what you're getting at.

Teacher: What are you seeing? [*Metacognitive question to assess what he is integrating.*]

Student: Thoughts could keep her from talking about her feelings. [*Now, he sees the defensive function of thoughts.*]

Teacher: So, would it make sense to block thoughts that take up space, so that the patient regains the space to talk about her feelings? [*Now that he sees how defenses take space away from feelings, can he understand the therapeutic task?*]

Student: Yes.

Teacher: What are you learning now about what takes space from the patient and how you can make space for the patient? [*Metacognitive question to assess what the student is integrating.*]

Student: I had thought I needed to allow space for everything. I didn't see how defenses don't allow space for the patient to talk about her feelings. [*Notice what he left out. That is what he has not integrated.*]

Teacher: And given that defenses take space away from the patient, as a therapist, how can you make space for her? [*Feedback-driven metacognitive question.*]

Student: I can block the thoughts and invite her to say more about her feelings.

Teacher: And how does that change your understanding of your therapeutic role? [*Metacognitive question to deepen the integration of new information.*]

Student: I just thought I needed to listen to everything coming in. But now I see I need to check if her words allow space for her feelings or take space away. [*The student is developing a basic understanding of his role as a therapist, which we can build on. And the static concept of space based on the assumption of no conflict shifts to a dynamic concept where defenses determine the amount of space.*]

Here, the student has a folk concept of space where he sits while the patient talks. For him, there is no need to analyze the function of anything the patient says. This folk concept of listening requires no clinical thinking because it assumes there is no unconscious conflict to think about. Through decision tree questions, the teacher helps the student analyze the function of the statements: do they make space for feelings or take up space? Once he can analyze the function of the patient's statements, he understands his therapeutic role in a new light. We make space for the patient by blocking defenses that take space away from her. Thus, space becomes a dynamic, clinical concept, which shrinks due to defenses or expands due to the therapist's interventions.

Monitoring Conceptual Change

If the student's clinical thinking does not change in the class or supervision session, her work will not change in the next therapy session. Therefore, we ask metacognitive questions to monitor whether students shift from the unconscious use of folk concepts to the conscious use of psychological concepts. "How does this change your understanding of defense work?"

Students cannot learn core ideas in psychotherapy unless their folk concepts change. For instance, suppose a patient complains about a husband who doesn't listen to her. When the student hears the latent content, it is painful to realize that the patient experiences the therapist as a poor listener, too. Unless the teacher helps the student bear this information, she will stop listening to latent content. But then she will not learn concepts such as "unconscious" or "transference" deeply. She may think the patient's husband is a poor listener. But her belief will prevent her from seeing that she is a poor listener. As a result, more patients will drop out. The teacher's prompts can help the student see the unconscious implications of the patient's words.

In the following example, a patient had quit therapy, and the therapist didn't understand why. "I thought we had a good alliance," she said. [*Folk concept: the alliance is "good" if the patient talks.*] She described her work with a severely disturbed patient. The patient had a dream in which a mass murderer was pursuing her.

Teacher: Suppose we listen from the perspective of the latent content. How might this dream symbolize her experience of you and the therapy? [*Inviting the student to listen to latent content: the unconscious symbolic meaning of the patient's words.*]

Student: I'm a mass murderer pursuing her?

Teacher: Although we both know you are a very kind person, yes, the patient may perceive you as if you are her killer. If so, how will she perceive your interventions? [*Inviting the student to think clinically using this listening perspective.*]

Student: As attempts to hurt her?

Teacher: And, given that, why would she quit? [*Inviting the patient to think clinically by using this listening perspective.*]

Student: To avoid a killer.

Teacher: Insofar as she perceived you as a killer, what interventions might have strengthened this belief? [*Inviting the patient to think clinically using this listening perspective.*]

Student: I kept trying to find out what was going on in her.

Teacher: How did you try to find out?

Student: I asked questions about her concerns and her history.

Teacher: If you represented a killer, how might she have experienced your questions? [*Inviting the patient to think clinically using this listening perspective.*]

Student: I get it. It's so weird. I thought we had a good alliance. [*She is beginning to think about her thinking and her previous bias.*]

Teacher: And what do you understand now? [*Metacognitive question to assess how new information changes old knowledge.*]

Student: She was afraid I would kill her. And that explains why she didn't want to come back when I called her.

Teacher: How does listening to the latent content change how you understand her? [*Metacognitive question to assess how new information changes old knowledge.*]

Student: I saw something I hadn't seen before. On the surface, I thought things were fine. But this lets me see what was going on in her. [*Her conditional knowledge has shifted. She understands when and why listening to latent content can be helpful.*]

Teacher: How does latent content change your understanding of how she experienced your interventions? [*Metacognitive question: how does new information change old knowledge?*]

Student: I thought they were okay. But now, I can see my questioning made her feel invaded. Oh. And she also talked about hunters.

Teacher: If we listen to the latent content, how does that change your understanding of her? [*Metacognitive question to assess how new information changes old knowledge.*]

Student: She experienced me as if I was hunting her.

Teacher: As if you were the hunter, and she was the prey. When we listen for latent content, how does your understanding of listening change? [*Metacognitive question to assess how new information changes old knowledge.*]

Student: I need to listen to what she says. But I can also listen to the symbolic meaning of the words to see how else she might be experiencing me and the therapy. [*She can think about and understand the importance of listening from multiple perspectives.*]

Teacher: And how is that different from how you were listening to her? [*Metacognitive question to assess how new information changes old knowledge.*]

Student: I listened to what she said but not the symbolic meaning.

Teacher: And when you listen in two ways to get more information, you can understand the patient more deeply.

The student was imprisoned because she could listen in only one way. By learning to listen to latent content, she began to hear a relational world she had never seen before. Listening in only one way made her the hostage of that lens, controlling what she could see.

After the class, the student confided, "This supervision was different for me. I thought it was about learning the interventions so I could use them afterward. But this time, I was learning to think."

Since she could listen only to the manifest content, her inability to hear latent content was the learning problem. Repeatedly analyzing the symbolic meanings of the patient's statements taught her how to listen to latent content. As she shifted from a folk concept to a clinical concept of listening, her capacity for clinical thinking deepened.

Likewise, her folk concept of a "good" alliance shifted. In egocentric thinking, she thought the alliance was good if it felt good to *her*. She paid attention to her experience rather than the patient's conscious and *unconscious* experience (Metz, Weisberg, & Weisberg, 2018; Prado, 2018). However, a good alliance depends on whether the *patient* experiences it as good. Through listening to latent content, she shifted from an egocentric to a relational concept of alliance.

The Role of Metacognitive Questions

I asked questions to help the student think about what she was learning and how her understanding was changing. And my follow-up questions facilitated her process of conceptual change. First, we teach a new concept or skill. Next, we invite the student to think about what she knows, what she is learning, and how her knowledge is changing. Metacognitive questions help students integrate new information with their prior knowledge. These questions also help us assess what the student is not integrating, so we know where to focus next.

Assessing Folk Concepts as Learning Problems

In the previous example, the student had a learning problem (Ekstein & Wallerstein, 1972). She thought she had a good alliance because she did not know how to listen to latent content. That was the most important thing to teach. I helped her unlearn folk concepts driving her unscientific thinking so that she could learn psychological concepts and skills for clinical thinking.

Sometimes, students' preconceptions are somewhat useful. Then, we can build on and develop them into scientific, psychological concepts. And when their ideas are incomplete, the teacher can fill in the gaps with new information (Chi, 2013). For instance, the student who learned more about sensitivity had a folk concept we could develop into a more complex clinical concept.

To facilitate conceptual change, teachers present evidence that conflicts with students' preconceptions. This gradually helps them adopt scientifically accurate information (Chinn & Malhotra, 2002). The instructor can do role-plays of therapy with students. For instance, the role-play with the student who wanted to be sensitive shows how to help students experience the limitations of a folk concept. Then, they become open to learning a new psychological concept, listening skill, or intervention.

If the teacher argues, the student may submit. But her misconception will continue to drive her work. Once she experiences the limitation of a bias, she can shift from intuitive notions to psychological concepts.

The instructor analyzes the student's preconceptions to understand the student's framework. Once she sees how it differs from the theory she is teaching, she can design a role-play so that the student experiences those differences and their effects (Shtulman, 2017). However, some misperceptions prevent clinical thinking, causing therapy to fail. Or the student may have a faulty model of human functioning. ("Just say no to drugs.")

To illustrate how to analyze biases, let's examine the phrase, "Just say no to drugs." This bias is not clinical thinking. But why? First, it rests on faulty assumptions. It assumes there are no unconscious *psychological* factors at work and no unconscious conflict. It assumes we pay attention *only* to the patient's conscious thoughts and feelings.

The statement does include a psychological concept: will. However, the statement assumes the patient has complete control as if no conflict interferes with his will. As a result of these assumptions, several ideas follow. "He didn't want to change." "He had no motivation." "He could have changed if he wanted to." Of course, those ideas make sense to the layperson who assumes that no unconscious psychological factors affect the patient's will. For the layperson, either the patient wanted to change, or he didn't.

Further, the student regards the statement as a conclusion to believe, not a hypothesis to test. Thus, the student does not analyze the patient's responses to change his hypothesis. Uninfluenced by the patient's responses, his thinking remains egocentric (Elder, 2019)— guided by his beliefs, not the patient's responses. We analyze the assumptions and biases driving the student's non-scientific thinking. Then, we can help the student think about his non-scientific thinking so that he can begin to think clinically.

Meanwhile, integrating new concepts and forms of reasoning reorganizes students' existing knowledge structures (Vosniadou, 2018). Thus, the teacher:

1 Teaches new concepts and skills.
2 Monitors how the student integrates new information into old knowledge.
3 Evaluates how the student uses psychological concepts for clinical thinking.

For instance, using folk concepts and biases results in narrative practices not grounded in a formal theory (Ratcliffe, 2007). Students may equate their socially supported story-telling activities with clinical thinking. For instance, they often speculate about patients or make things up like they did in their background. As a result, students feel overconfident: "I know what this means!" Here is a common example.

Student: His parents can't tolerate his having a separate mind. [*A common story-telling strategy among laypersons: treat an assumption about others as a truth.*]
Teacher: Have you met his parents? [*Question about a folk assumption.*]
Student: No.
Teacher: Then how would you know? [*Question about a folk assumption.*]
Student: It seems that way to me.
Teacher: Yes. Your thought seems true to you. That makes sense since you had it. But have you met his parents so you could know if your thought is true?
Student: No.
Teacher: It is a plausible hypothesis, but is there any way you can test it? [*Teaching a principle of clinical thinking: we test hypotheses. The student has offered an invalid assumption, not a hypothesis. So, I use the word "hypothesis" to help him remove his layperson hat and put on his clinical thinking hat.*]
Student: No.
Teacher: So, let's step back for a moment and see what we have learned. In social conversation, we often speculate about people. But in clinical thinking, we do something different. What differences did you just learn about? [*Metacognitive question to assess what the student is integrating.*]
Student: I shouldn't assume something is true about someone unless I have met them.

Teacher: Right. And what else?

Student: I don't know. [*The student forgot one other important element. What he forgets, he will not integrate. So we give him a prompt.*]

Teacher: And when you form an opinion, do we believe it? [*Can he remember that an opinion is not a fact?*]

Student: No. I have to test it.

Teacher: So rather than treat it as a belief or a truth, we treat it as a ... [*Half-question.*]

Student: Hypothesis. [*Using the word "hypothesis" helps the student shift to clinical thinking.*]

Teacher: You had a thought about people you have not met. And you assumed it was true. Then you learned how we treat a thought, not as a fact but as a hypothesis to test. We compare a hypothesis with evidence from the patient. Without evidence, we can't test the hypothesis. How is clinical thinking different from your previous way of thinking? [*Metacognitive question: can he think about his thinking? What is he integrating?*]

The teacher helps the student see the limitations of a story-telling strategy. And the student learns that his belief is not a fact. Further, he learns that we base clinical thinking on evidence from the patient, not fantasies in our minds. This process facilitates conceptual change.

To understand conceptual change, we can use framework theory (Vosniadou, 2018). Beginning students have already formed a naïve psychology based on their experiences and cultural beliefs. This naïve psychology "forms a loose but relatively coherent explanatory system, a framework theory" (Vosniadou, 2018, p. 18).

When learning psychotherapy, the student's framework changes. She lets go of some biases. Her preconceptions change. And she learns new concepts. Further, she learns new forms of reasoning. She assesses whether evidence from the patient supports her hypotheses. And by learning from the patient, she discovers a new relational epistemology: patients' responses change her thinking. As a result, how she listens, thinks about, and relates to people changes. No wonder change takes time!

Why Are Misconceptions So Robust?

Some misconceptions resolve through proper instruction. However, other misconceptions persist even when teachers focus on them (Chi, 2005). Why? Many misconceptions mis-categorize the ontology of a concept. In other words, when something exists, what is its nature: its ontology? Have we conceived it correctly? An *ontological shift* is necessary for the student to overcome a misconception (Chi, 2005).

To illustrate an ontological shift, let us examine depression. Students often refer to depression as if it is an *entity*, a thing the patient *has*. They conflate the ontologies of *entities* and *processes*. Depression is not a thing. It emerges as the result of an ongoing *process* of defenses constantly creating it. If depression is an entity that exists, we can do nothing to make it disappear. But if it emerges from a process, we can intervene to interrupt the process, so that it no longer creates depression.

Perhaps the most common robust misconception in psychotherapy is the term "diagnosis." The DSM-V or the ICD-11 diagnostic categories describe symptoms. For instance, "major depression, recurrent" refers to a list of symptoms. However, describing symptoms does not explain their cause. A genuine diagnosis explains the *process* that causes those symptoms over time. Then, we can treat the cause. Therefore, when teaching assessment, psychotherapy teachers help students understand symptoms as *products* of continuous psychological *processes*. Then, we help students shift their attention to those *processes* that are active outside and inside the therapy session. Any psychotherapy model based on a psychological theory focuses on the processes causing symptoms. Psychodynamic therapists focus on dynamic forces and conflicts causing symptoms. Behavior therapists teach chain behavior analysis. Cognitive behavioral therapists teach causal analysis.

Let's look at another question that reveals a folk assumption with a mistaken ontology.

Student: Isn't there a danger of taking away the patient's defenses?
Teacher: That's an interesting question. Suppose I hand Jane my wallet. [*I take it out of my pocket and hand it to Jane.*] Jane could take away my wallet, couldn't she? Why?
Students: Because it is a thing.
Teacher: Right. It is a material object. Now, can Jane take away my ability to intellectualize? [*Students discuss back and forth, puzzled by the question.*] [*I invite them to notice how they treat a concept, defense, as if it is a physical object. Metacognition about their concrete thinking.*]
Jim: No.
Teacher: Why can't Jane take away my ability to intellectualize?
John: Because it is a behavior?
Teacher: Exactly. I've had twenty years of therapy, and I can still intellectualize any time I want to!
[*Students laugh.*]
Teacher: How many of you have been in therapy?
[*Students raise their hands.*]
Teacher: Were your therapists able to take away your defenses?
[*Class laughs.*]

Teacher: No. Even if we could, we have no right to take away anyone's defenses. Second, we can't take away defenses because they are strategies for handling feelings. And no one can take a strategy away from you. How does the idea of strategies change your understanding of defenses? [*A metacognitive question assesses what the students are integrating and not integrating.*]

A concrete question opens a beautiful learning opportunity. Students learned that a defense is not a thing, *an entity*, but a strategy we can use. Once we correct that incorrect ontology, students can shift from a folk concept to a psychological concept of defense. Otherwise, they will avoid defense work if they believe they are "taking something" from the patient. The "stupid" question often reveals the learning problem to address.

Some folk misconceptions involve the concept of *causality*. For instance, "The patient got depressed after she was fired six months ago." The student thinks the depression occurs due to an event in the past rather than processes in the present. When her attention is riveted on a past event (Grotzer, 2012), she cannot pay attention to the unconscious defenses causing her depression now.

Science students learn about non-obvious or invisible processes involving causality such as gravity and air pressure. So do beginning psychotherapy students. For instance, the unconscious *function* of a statement reveals a non-obvious cause. The latent content discloses the patient's unconscious perception of therapy. "Is it possible that there are things going on around us—even causes and effects—that we cannot see?" (Grotzer, 2012, p. 110). Students learn to perceive invisible causes in science and psychotherapy.

Principle: *To understand the patient's symptoms, we analyze the psychological processes causing them.*

Misconceptions and Causality in Psychotherapy

We engage in clinical thinking to discover what causes the patient's presenting problems. The beginning student thinks about causality but in linear, agentic terms. "This patient did not want to get better. So he stayed depressed." This student assumes that symptoms result only from the patient's conscious agency. For him, there is one variable (the patient's refusal) and one outcome (failure). However, linear, agentic causality does not apply to most clinical problems. Thus, we teach different patterns of causation (Grotzer, 2012) to broaden students' understanding of causes and effects.

Let's take, for example, the expert therapist. She might wonder what unconscious defenses cause the patient's depression. She thinks in terms of a *non-agentic form of causality*. For instance, what unconscious defenses interfere with the patient's conscious agency? What unconscious schemas or transferences (relational patterns) damage the patient's relationships? Once we consider unconscious factors, we no longer think of causality only in terms of a conscious agent. The layperson who thinks in terms of conscious determinism——"Just say no to drugs"——will not see the unconscious factors at work. The expert also looks for unconscious factors that might determine the patient's behaviors, interfering with his conscious agency.

Suppose the supervisor sees a case where the therapeutic relationship causes the problem. For example, when the patient becomes passive, the therapist becomes more active. Then, the patient becomes more passive, triggering the therapist to be more active. They enact a passive/active feedback loop. We cannot say the patient is the cause, nor can we say it is the therapist. They both contribute to a cycle; hence, we see *cyclical causality*. Their feedback loop perpetuates the status quo, leading to a stuck therapy. However, the supervisor can help the student see how she contributes to the feedback loop. Then, she can ask herself, "What can I do differently to stop reinforcing the patient's passivity?"

We saw a case where the patient projected the image of a hunter onto the therapist. That case was a form of *spiraling causality*, a feedback loop where her symptoms continued to worsen. She believed her projection, her anxiety spiraled, so she projected more, increasing her anxiety. Another example would be a therapist who focuses primarily on defenses. Each time the therapist addresses a defense, the patient feels judged, and her depression spirals downward (A. Freud, 1936). *Spiraling causality* is essential to perceive because it can lead to rapidly escalating anxiety or depression, then dropout.

Often, we help students see *domino causality*, where a sequence of events triggers symptoms or presenting problems. In behavior therapy, chain behavior analysis detects this form of causality. Here, an effect becomes a cause. For instance, a relationship triggers feelings (result) in the patient. Feelings (a result) trigger (cause) anxiety. Anxiety (a result) triggers (causes) defenses. And defenses (a result) (cause) presenting problems and symptoms. When effects become causes, students may have trouble seeing the entire pattern. For instance, the student may see how a defense of self-attack causes the patient to become depressed. But he may not see the rest of the dominos——the stimulus, feelings, and anxiety that preceded the defense. Only if the therapist observes the entire causal chain can he understand when to intervene, interrupt the domino causality, and prevent a misalliance with the patient. Further, when the therapist perceives the pattern, he can intervene earlier in the sequence, preventing symptom formation in the session.

The student, unaware of the kind of causal thinking he uses, cannot think about it. Thus, we teach him to think about the form of causality he uses to understand the patient. Then, we can help him see the evidence that a linear, agentic form of causality omits.

In our causal reasoning, the information we think is relevant "determines what we attend to and what we don't" (Grotzer, 2012, p. 32). Consider the layperson who perceives only linear, agentic causality. His perspective will limit the information he attends to. As a result, he "may not seek mechanisms to explain complex phenomena that [he is] unaware of" (Grotzer, 2012, p. 32). For instance, the student who thought she had a good alliance saw nothing to analyze until her patient quit therapy. When we understand different forms of causality, we can direct our attention to specific kinds of information and become aware of causal mechanisms we had not seen. Thus, teaching alternative forms of causality helps students recognize forms of causation they hadn't seen so that they can intervene more effectively.

Common Problems with Critical Thinking in the Field

Therapists are often not taught to think critically. As a result, beginning students may not detect common thinking errors or cognitive biases (Garb, 1998; Elder, 2019; Kahneman & Tversky, 1996). Let us review common mistakes, biases, and assumptions (Meehl, 1973, 2006; Ruscio, 2006).

The Barnum Effect: Make a superficial statement that is true of nearly everyone. Then, state it as if it is important and unique to a specific patient (Meehl, 2006). While this is common among palm readers, therapist examples include "This patient suffered from traumas," "She has self-esteem issues," "His problem is anxiety." True, perhaps, but vague and general, thus trivial and non-informative.

Multiple Napoleons fallacy: "So what if he thinks he's Napoleon? It feels real to him." A therapist differentiates reality from delusion to assess reality testing. If you think there is a man on the moon, and I say it is a geological formation, one of us is wrong. It is a waste of time to point out that a patient perceives his delusion as real. That's what a delusion is: belief in a false perception. The statement "It is real to him" is philosophically either trivial or false (Meehl, 1973). Further, it distracts us from assessing the loss of reality testing, its extent, and its causes.

The spun glass theory of the mind: Sometimes therapists treat minor events as major traumas. They believe humans are made of spun glass. However, this belief ignores patients' resilience and ability to recover. When we assume a patient cannot recover, despair becomes a substitute for clinical thought.

Anti-biology bias: Some psychotherapists react negatively to biological contributors to abnormal behavior. Thus, they oppose medication, dispute the role of genetics, and always oppose ECT. Here, bias substitutes for clinical thinking. Likewise, clinicians who rely on only biological explanations reveal their anti-psychological bias—biological reductionism (Kinderman, 2005).

Pseudo-science: Practitioners make unsubstantiated claims for treatments with pseudo-scientific names, rationalized with psychobabble. Take, for instance, The Brain SuperCharger. The Brain SuperCharger is an audio recording. It "alters consciousness opening a doorway into your subconscious to rewire negative self-sabotaging beliefs" (Thyer & Pignotti, 2015, pp. 56–57). Here, belief in pseudo-scientific fantasies substitutes for scientific thinking about clinical data.

A description is not an explanation: A student describes a symptom but not its cause. For instance, she offers a label for the patient, "major depression, recurrent." However, when the teacher asks what causes the patient's symptoms, the student does not know. Therefore, she cannot treat the cause (Bateson, 2000; McWilliams, 2021; Verhaeghe, 2019). What we call "diagnosis" in the psychotherapy field is a misnomer. The so-called "diagnosis" only describes symptoms. However, describing patients' symptoms does not explain their cause.

Students often cannot differentiate between clinical and unscientific forms of thinking. As a result, belief, bias, and pseudo-scientific fantasies may substitute for clinical thought. Then, students cannot diagnose the cause of psychological symptoms.

The myth that thinking does not require a theory or concepts

Students often believe that theory and concepts are not necessary for thinking. As a result, they don't understand the function, strengths, and limitations of concepts.

A supervisor was teaching the concept of conflict. So she asked a student, "Where is the patient's response on the triangle of conflict? Did she offer a feeling, did she become anxious, or did she offer a defense?"

Student: Are there only three options? [*The student feels confined. She does not understand that each concept limits what we look at so that we can focus on specific patterns.*]

Teacher: Yes, there only three options when we look at the patient's response through the lens of conflict. If we look at his statement through the lens of schema, there are other options. And if we look at his statement through the lens of chain behavior analysis, there are still others. Every concept is a tool of perception. It allows us to focus on certain things and not others. Consider other tools for perception. Glasses help you read a book, but you need a telescope to see the stars or an electron microscope to see a molecule. Each tool helps, yet we could not use an electron microscope to read a book. The same is true of concepts. Every concept allows us to see specific patterns and not others. That's why we need many concepts to look at what patients say and do through multiple perspectives.

Student: But looking at the patient this way feels so limiting.

Teacher: Of course! Every concept limits what we examine to direct our attention to patterns we ordinarily wouldn't see. An electron microscope eliminates almost everything we can see with the eyes, so we can study a cell. Likewise, concepts help us perceive patterns we couldn't see before. Shall we keep working with the concept of conflict so you can learn to see this pattern that was invisible before?

The beginning therapist has spent a lifetime thinking by using concepts unconsciously. Thus, she is not aware of the concepts she uses and how they direct her attention and limit what she can perceive. When she learns psychological concepts, she discovers how concepts direct our attention. And she learns how each concept both limits and expands our awareness. Now she uses psychological concepts consciously to perceive different patterns so folk concepts no longer unconsciously determine what she can see.

Common Substitutes for Teaching Clinical Thinking

While students may engage in uncritical thinking, teachers and supervisors can too. The following examples illustrate uncritical thinking that my students or I have heard in class or supervision.

"Trust the process." Several questions arise: 1) What do we mean by "process"? 2) What process is taking place? 3) Is this process helping the patient or not? 4) If not, how can we change it? The term "process" refers to the sequence of the patient's associations. As we listen to that sequence, can the patient elaborate on a painful topic? Or do defenses inhibit the patient? No one should trust a process that is not working. Blind trust is magical thinking, not clinical thinking. So, we help the student assess the process moment by moment to see whether it leads to illness or health.

"You need to log more hours." The supervisee is told to trust time, not expertise. There is nothing magical about time. The question is: what are the therapist and patient doing in the time they have? Is the patient getting better or not? If not, why not? Trusting time is magical thinking. Assessing progress is clinical thinking.

"You need to build more trust." But how? Is the patient interacting with a projection? Is he using a wall of detachment and doubt? Or is he recognizing a problem in the clinician? What skills does the student need? Here, a statement, "build trust," tells the student what to do but not how to do it.

"Your love will melt defenses." Here, omnipotent denial substitutes for clinical thinking. The therapist's love supposedly can erase the patient's difficulties. "All you need is love." A magical wish denies the need for real skills. Therapy is hard to do. Thus, we will always have simplistic pseudo-answers for genuine questions. However, if we recognize what clinical thinking is, we can help students learn to do it.

Moving from Unconscious Assumptions to the Conscious Use of Psychological Concepts

We could say that the beginning student does not control his thinking. Instead, unconscious assumptions, biases, and preconceptions control what he can perceive and, thus, think about. In clinical thinking, we try to be conscious of the concepts we use so that we can control our thinking. We try to recognize an assumption *as an assumption*, an inference *as an inference*, and a conclusion *as a conclusion* (Norris & Phillips, 2012; Olson, 1994). Thus, we help students consciously use psychological concepts and think about what those concepts allow us to perceive.

Summary

Psychotherapy education and supervision emancipates the student from former biases and assumptions, so they no longer dominate his thinking and feeling. It is not the teacher's task to indoctrinate the student into a favored belief but to help him recognize and free himself from unconscious beliefs so that he can become a thinker. The beginning therapist does not necessarily know what clinical listening is. He does not know the clinical concepts we use to analyze what people say and do. He does not know how to compare hypotheses with evidence, or what that evidence might be. As a result, he may believe his thoughts rather than test them. "If I think it, that makes it so."

When unquestioned biases direct our thinking, we cannot think about our assumptions or how they shape our thinking. The layperson often believes his intuitive feelings are a better source of knowledge than evidence from the patient. At worst, he may care less about facts than preserving his biases. As a result, he will not understand what drives patients' suffering.

Thus, we identify unquestioned assumptions to help students notice their biases and preconceptions. Unlearning allows new learning. As they experience the limitations of their misconceptions and think about them, they enter a new world of clinical thinking.

However, letting go of old ideas and learning new ones can be disruptive. It feels strange and even wrong to listen, think, and intervene in new ways. Anxiety rises when students let go of old habits to learn new skills. So, let us see how to help students cope with the anxiety caused by conceptual and personal change.

Questions for the Teacher and Supervisor to Ask about the Student

1   What does the student see, and what doesn't she see?
2   What folk concepts and misconceptions interfere with what the student can see?
3   What assumptions are driving the student's interventions?
4   How might you structure a role-play, so that the student experiences the limitations of her assumptions?
5   What biases and assumptions do you need to unlearn about teaching and supervision?

References

Abbass, A. (2015). *Reaching through resistance*. Kansas City, Mo.: Seven Leaves Press.

Barlow, D., & Farchione, T. (Eds.). (2017). *Applications of the unified protocol for transdiagnostic treatment of emotional disorders*. New York: Oxford University Press.

Bateson, G. (2000). *Steps to an ecology of mind: Collected essays in anthropology, psychiatry, evolution, and epistemology*. Chicago: University of Chicago Press.

Chi, M., Bassok, M., Lewis, M., Reimann, P., & Glaser, R. (1989). Self-explanation: How students study and use examples in learning to solve problems. *Cognitive Science, 13*, 145–182.

Chi, M. (2005). Commonsense conceptions of emergent process: Why some misconceptions are robust. *The Journal of the Learning Sciences, 14*(2), 161–199.

Chi, M. (2013). Two kinds and four sub-types of misconceived knowledge: Ways to change it, and the learning outcomes. In S. Vosniadou (Ed.), *International handbook of research on conceptual change* (pp. 49–70). New York: Routledge.

Chinn, C., & Malhotra, A. (2002). Children's responses to anomalous scientific data: How is conceptual change impeded? *Journal of Research in Science Teaching, 35*, 623–635.

Churchland, P. M. (1998). Folk psychology. In P. M. Churchland & P. S. Churchland, *On the Contrary: Critical Essays 1987–1997* (pp. 3–16). Cambridge, Mass.: MIT Press.

Damasio, A. (2000). *The feeling of what happens: Body and emotion in the making of consciousness*. New York: Mariner Books.

Davison, W. T., Bristol, C., & Pray, M. (1986). Turning aggression on the self: A study of psychoanalytic process. *The Psychoanalytic Quarterly, 55*(2), 273–295.

Davison, W. T., Pray, M., & Bristol, C. (1990). Mutative interpretation and close process monitoring in a study of psychoanalytic process. *The Psychoanalytic Quarterly, 59*(4), 599–628.

Ekman, P. (2003). *Emotions revealed: Recognizing faces and feelings to improve communication and emotional life.* New York: Times Books.

Ekstein, R., & Wallerstein, R. (1972). *The teaching and learning of psychotherapy* (2nd ed.). New York: International Universities Press.

Elder, L. (2019). *Liberating the mind: Overcoming sociocentric thought and egocentric tendencies.* Lanham, Md.: Rowman and Littlefield.

Fletcher, G. (1995). *The scientific credibility of folk psychology.* New York: Lawrence Erlbaum.

Frederickson, J. (1999). *Psychodynamic psychotherapy: Listening from multiple perspectives.* New York: Routledge.

Frederickson, J. (2013). *Co-creating change: Effective dynamic therapy techniques.* Kansas City, Mo.: Seven Leaves Press.

Frederickson, J. (2020). *Co-creating safety: Healing the fragile patient.* Kensington, Md.: Seven Leaves Press.

Freud, A. (1936). *The ego and the mechanisms of defense.* New York: Norton.

Freud, S. (1961a). The ego and the id. In J. Strachey (Ed. and Trans.), *The standard edition of the complete psychological works of Sigmund Freud, Vol. 19* (pp. 3–66). New York: W.W. Norton. (Original work published 1923)

Freud, S. (1961b). Inhibitions, symptoms, and anxiety. In J. Strachey (Ed. and Trans.), *The standard edition of the complete psychological works of Sigmund Freud, Vol. 20* (pp. 75–175). New York: W.W. Norton. (Original work published 1926)

Garb, H. (1998). *Studying the clinician: Judgment research and psychological assessment.* Washington, D.C.: American Psychological Association.

Goldwater, M., & Schalk, L. (2016). Relational categories as a bridge between cognitive and educational research. *Psychological Bulletin, 142*(7), 729–757.

Gray, P. (1994). *The ego and the analysis of defense.* New York: Aronson.

Grotzer, T. (2012). *Learning causality in a complex world: Understandings of consequence.* Lanham, Md.: R & L Education.

Gutman, A. (1979). Misconceptions of psychology and performance in the introductory course. *Teaching of Psychology, 6*(3), 159–161.

Hartman, H. (2001). Developing students' metacognitive knowledge and strategies. In H. Hartman (Ed.), *Metacognition in learning and instruction: Theory, research, and practice* (pp. 33–68). Dordrecht, Netherlands: Kluwer Academic Publishers.

Havens, L. (1986). *Making contact: The uses of language in psychotherapy.* Cambridge, Mass.: Harvard University Press.

Hiebert, J., & Lefevre, P. (1986). Conceptual and procedural knowledge in mathematics: An introductory analysis. In J. Hiebert (Ed.), *Conceptual and procedural knowledge: The case of mathematics* (pp. 1–27). Mahwah, N.J: Lawrence Erlbaum Associates, Inc.

Janig, W. (2008). *The integrative function of the autonomic nervous system.* Cambridge, UK: Cambridge University Press.

Kahneman, D., & Tversky, A. (1996). On the reality of cognitive illusions. *Psychological Review*, 103(3), 582–591, discussion 592–596. https://doi.org/10.1037/0033-295X.103.3.582

Kernberg, O. (2001). Object relations, affects, and drives: Toward a new synthesis. *Psychoanalytic Inquiry*, 21(5), 604–619.

Kinderman, P. (2005). A psychological model of mental disorder. *Harvard Review of Psychiatry*, 13(4), 206–217.

Kottler, J., & Balkin, R. (2020). *Myths, misconceptions, and invalid assumptions of counseling and psychotherapy*. Oxford: Oxford University Press.

Langs, R. (1989a). *The technique of psychoanalytic psychotherapy: Vol. 1. Initial contact: Theoretical framework: Understanding the patient's communications: The therapist's interventions*. New York: Aronson.

Langs, R. (1989b). *The technique of psychoanalytic psychotherapy: Vol. 2. Responses to interventions: Patient-therapist relationship: Phases of psychotherapy*. New York: Aronson.

LeDoux, J. (1998). *The emotional brain: The mysterious underpinnings of emotional life*. New York: Simon and Schuster.

Lemov, D. (2021). *Teach like a champion 3.0*. New York: Jossey-Bass.

Lundholm, C. (2018). Conceptual change and the complexity of learning. In T. G. Amin & O. Levrini (Eds.), *Converging perspectives on conceptual change: Mapping an emerging paradigm in the learning sciences* (pp. 34–42). New York: Routledge/Taylor & Francis Group.

Marsh, E., & Eliseev, E. (2019). Correcting student errors and misconceptions. In J. Dunlosky, & K. Rawson (Eds.), *The Cambridge handbook of cognition and education* (pp. 437–459). Cambridge, UK: Cambridge University Press.

Matte Blanco, I. (1975). *The unconscious as infinite sets*. London: Karnac.

McWilliams, N. (2021). *Psychoanalytic diagnosis: Understanding personality structure in the clinical process* (2nd ed.). New York: Guilford Press.

Meehl, P. (1973). *Psychodiagnosis: Selected papers*. Minneapolis, Minn.: University of Minnesota Press.

Meehl, P. (2006). *A Paul Meehl reader: Essays on the practice of scientific psychology*. Mahwah, N.J.: Lawrence Erlbaum Associates.

Metz, S., Weisberg, D., & Weisberg, M. (2018). Non-scientific criteria for belief sustain non-scientific beliefs. *Cognitive Science*, 42(5), 1477–1503.

Norris, S. & Phillips, L. (2012). Reading science: How a naïve view of reading hinders so much else. In A. Zohar & Y. Dori (Eds.), *Metacognition in science education: Trends in current research* (pp. 37–56). New York: Springer.

Ogden, T. (1992). *Projective identification and psychotherapeutic technique*. New York: Jason Aronson.

Olson, D. (1994). *The world on paper*. Cambridge, UK: Cambridge University Press.

Paniagua, C. (1991). Patient's surface, clinical surface, and workable surface. *Journal of the American Psychoanalytic Association*, 39, 669–685.

Porges, S. (2011). *The polyvagal theory: Neurophysiological foundations of emotions, attachment, communication, and self-regulation*. New York: Norton.

Prado, C. (Ed.). (2018). *America's post-truth phenomenon: When feelings and opinions trump facts and evidence*. Santa Barbara, Calif.: Praeger.

Racker, H. (1968). *Transference and countertransference*. New York: International Universities Press.

Ratcliffe, M. (2007). *Rethinking commonsense psychology: A critique of folk psychology, theory of mind and simulation*. London: Palgrave MacMillan.

Robertson, D., Biaggioni, I., Burnstock, G., Low, P., & Paton, J. (2004). *Primer on the autonomic nervous system*. Amsterdam: Elsevier.

Ruscio, J. (2006). *Critical thinking in psychology: Separating sense from nonsense*. Boston: Wadsworth Cengage Learning.

Saposnik, G., Redelmeier, D., Ruff, C. C., & Tobler, P. N. (2016). Cognitive biases associated with medical decisions: A systematic review. *BMC Medical Informatics and Decision Making, 16*, Article 138.

diSessa, A. (2022). A history of conceptual change research. In R. Sawyer (Ed.), *The Cambridge handbook of the learning sciences* (3rd ed., pp. 114–133). Cambridge, UK: Cambridge University Press.

Shtulman, A. (2017). *Scienceblind: Why our intuitive theories about the world are so often wrong*. New York: Basic Books.

Solms, M. (2021). *The hidden spring: Journey to the source of consciousness*. New York: Norton.

Tansey, M., & Burke, W. (1995). *Understanding countertransference: From projective identification to empathy*. New York: Routledge.

Taylor, A., & Kowalski, P. (2014). Student misconceptions: Where do they come from and what can we do? In V. Benassi, C. Overson, & C. Hakal (Eds.), *Applying science of learning in education: Infusing psychological science into the curriculum* (pp. 259–273). Society for the Teaching of Psychology. http://teachpsych.org/ebooks/asle2014/index.php

Thyer, B., Pignotti, A., & Monica, G. (2015). *Science and pseudoscience in social work practice*. New York: Springer.

Verhaeghe, P. (2019). *On being normal and other disorders: A manual for clinical psychodiagnostics*. New York: Routledge.

Vosniadou, S. (2018). Initial and scientific understandings and the problem of conceptual change. In T. Amin & O. Levrini (Eds.), *Converging perspectives on conceptual change: Mapping the emerging paradigm in the learning sciences* (pp. 17–25). New York: Routledge.

Zohar, A. & Dori, Y. (Eds.). (2012). *Metacognition in science education: Trends in current research*. New York: Springer.

Chapter 4

Positive Disintegration: Why Learning Triggers Anxiety

Jon Frederickson

Positive Disintegration: The Inevitable Result of Good Psychotherapy Teaching

New ideas dissolve our old way of thinking. Disintegration of old knowledge is positive because it allows us to integrate new information. However, it does not always feel positive to the student. Instead, it may feel confusing, wrong, or even dangerous. In fact, the student may feel personally threatened when her old way of thinking is changing. Thus, teachers normalize the repeated phases of positive disintegration (Dabrowski, 2017)—the journey of learning through living as therapists.

Student: This new intervention doesn't feel right.
Teacher: What doesn't feel right about it? [*Inviting the student to think about her learning process.*]
Student: It's so different. It doesn't feel natural to me or authentic.
Teacher: Of course! Since a habit feels so natural, anything different feels unnatural. Previously, you did reflection. Now you are learning to listen to latent content. Then you can discover the patient's perceptions that keep the treatment stuck. You wanted to learn something new. And I'm offering the new knowledge you want. But integrating this new information and new way of listening doesn't feel natural. Your old habit of reflection feels natural because it's familiar. And listening to latent content is entirely unfamiliar. [*Normalizing the discomfort of positive disintegration.*] How does listening to latent content differ from reflection?
Student: I feel like I want to argue. [*New information conflicts with old knowledge. But the student mistakes her inner conflict for an outer conflict with a teacher.*]
Teacher: Of course! Old knowledge argues with new information. New knowledge never precisely fits what you know. How is old knowledge arguing with new information right now? [*Help the*

DOI: 10.4324/9781003488637-4

student observe her learning process and struggle to integrate new knowledge. Help her see that there is no struggle between you and her. Instead, the tension occurs between what she knows and what she is learning.]

Student: I don't feel comfortable.

Teacher: Of course! We feel uncomfortable when old knowledge integrates new information. How do you experience that discomfort? [*Validate the discomfort of positive disintegration to help the student bear the anxiety of integrating new learning.*]

Students shift from misconceptions to use psychological concepts for clinical thinking. Instead of relying on assumptions and fantasies in their minds, they depend on evidence from patients. Rather than react habitually, they learn to intervene strategically. Their folk knowledge disintegrates. Learning clinical skills takes students out of their previous habits.

There is no such thing as effortless learning when mastering new skills in any field. Actively learning skills is always challenging. But why is it so hard for psychotherapists?

Learning a new stance for a serve in tennis changes where you put your feet. But becoming a therapist transforms how you listen, think, and relate to patients. And these changes can feel like a threat to the student's identity.

Students enter training as amateur psychologists using a folk psychology. Learning different clinical thinking and intervention skills takes them outside their comfort zone. Students' comfort zones have boundaries created by their preconceptions, habits, and biases. *There is no comfort zone in excellent learning* because it always takes us out of our habits (Janet Metcalfe, in Boser, 2017). Thus, teachers and supervisors address and normalize students' anxiety caused by undergoing the process of conceptual change.

Table 4.1 Comfort zone, learning zone, and shut down zone

Comfort Zone	Learning Zone	Shut Down Zone
The student is comfortable using her habits, biases, and preconceptions. No deep learning occurs.	The student tolerates anxiety as she lets go of biases and preconceptions to learn new things contrary to her previous habits. Deep learning occurs.	The student's excessive anxiety or shame prevents deep learning. Compliance, tuning out, or opposition occur as coping strategies. The student learns to oppose learning.

If the teacher does not regulate students' anxiety, they will resist the change they seek. And they will revert to their habitual reactions, failing to integrate new learning. Some will say they are not comfortable. Others will say, "This doesn't feel like me." Why?

The beginning therapist may have a relatively concrete view of himself. Teachers point out habitual styles of listening, thinking, or relating. But the student may reply, "This is who I am." He equates his habitual patterns of thinking and listening with who he is. However, he is not a listening perspective, a concept, or a habit. Thus, we help the student differentiate himself from his folk concepts and biases. And we support him during these periods of disruptive conceptual change (Owens et al., 2020).

Rumelhart & Norman (1978) proposed three modes of learning: accretion, structuring, and tuning. Through accretion, students add new information to the existing cognitive structure. Tuning refers to the ways that students refine and sharpen a cognitive structure based on new information. Structuring occurs when students replace a cognitive structure due to new information that shows the old one to be inadequate. Although adding to or refining a concept can trigger some anxiety, restructuring—replacing folk ideas and concepts—causes the most distress. And replacing ideas and concepts occurs most frequently during the initial phase of learning psychotherapy. Learning arouses feelings (Zohar & Barzilai, 2015). If we help students observe the feelings aroused by learning, they can regulate themselves and learn. That's why we pay close attention to positive disintegration.

To summarize, learning psychotherapy involves conceptual change, which triggers emotions and anxiety because the student's previous identity as a listener dissolves. Therefore, the supervisor monitors and regulates anxiety in the learning process (Alonso & Rutan, 1988). Otherwise, reactions to the anxiety can prevent further learning. To regulate anxiety, we can encourage a culture of compassion in class and supervision.

Principle: Good psychotherapy training changes the student as a person. This growth arouses anxiety. Normalize this process so that students can bear the disintegration of change while integrating new learning.

Culture of Compassion

A culture of compassion supports students' self-esteem while engaging in the learning task that threatens it. How do we create a culture of compassion? Invite it.

Inviting a culture of compassion: "I'm going to invite you to join me in creating a culture of compassion. In this class, each of you will reveal your work through videotaped cases. And you will reveal yourselves, your strengths, your weaknesses, what you know, and what you don't know. To do this, we must agree to be compassionate with one another as fellow learners. I'm going to ask you to raise your hands now. How many of you are willing to be compassionate with your class members when they make mistakes? Good. Here is the hard question. How many of you are willing to try to be compassionate with yourselves when you make mistakes? Good. And finally, how many of you are willing to help your classmates be compassionate with themselves when they make mistakes? Good. We need to co-create a culture of compassion. Here, we will learn psychotherapy skills. And while learning, all of us will make mistakes. Making mistakes is how we gain expertise.

Next, raise your hands if you make mistakes in therapy. Good. I'm glad to know I am in the right group. All of us make mistakes. The only reason I am good at pointing out mistakes is because I have made them. And I have made them many more times than you! The best therapists succeed only about 70–80% of the time, so even they are making mistakes.

We make mistakes when learning any complex skill like psychotherapy. They are necessary for learning. When we make a mistake, we can learn: "Hmm. What was the problem in my assessment that led to this mistake? What didn't I see? Now that I see it, how does it change my assessment? Given this new assessment, how could I intervene now?" Mistakes help us grow; they tell us what to learn. So, are you willing to be compassionate with each other when you make mistakes in this class? Okay. Now, we can begin. Welcome to our club: the mistake-makers."

Mistakes: Why Learning Triggers Anxiety

When students passively listen to a lecture, their lack of understanding can remain hidden. However, actively answering decision tree questions or doing skill-building exercises exposes students' mistakes. Now, students *experience* what they do not know and cannot do. And making mistakes in class through role-plays, skill-building exercises, and analyses of one's videotaped work raises students' anxiety, shame, and guilt (Alonso & Rutan, 1988; Hahn, 2001).

Normalize mistakes to regulate the anxiety and shame caused by perfectionism (Arkowitz, 2001). Remind the group of their task: to learn by making mistakes within a culture of compassion (Talbot, 1995). First, we get it wrong. Then, we get it wrong a few more times. And then, we get it right.

Student: I made a mistake.

Teacher: [*raising hands*] How many of you make mistakes? [*Everyone raises their hands and laughs.*] Okay. It sounds like we are in the right group. I was afraid I might be the only mistake-maker here. [*Deactivate shame.*] Let's analyze the patient's response so we can figure out how to intervene. [*Return to the learning task.*]

When the student becomes aware of a mistake, guilt will often arise. If she has trouble tolerating her guilt, she may criticize herself or fear others will. At that point, she wards off judgment rather than integrates learning. To block that process, interrupt as soon as the student says she made a mistake, as in the example above. The teacher's statement interrupts any self-judgment by the student. And it deactivates her projection of judgment onto the teacher. The sequence to avoid is a mistake, guilt, and self-criticism. Offer compassion after the mistake, before she can criticize herself. Then she can learn.

Also, when a student makes a mistake, invite her to intervene again with her new knowledge. Practice the skill with her until she masters it. I will never forget a student with whom I persisted for twenty minutes until she mastered a skill. Then she burst into tears, "No one was ever this patient with me before." What is patience? The ability to be with the student as she is. So, persist until the student experiences mastery.

Making mistakes is how we learn. Teachers should mention their mistakes and what they learned from them. Ideally, teachers show videos of their work with patients and point out their errors. Or they ask students to find the teacher's error and analyze why it is a mistake. This deactivates idealization of the teacher and the therapy model. Plus, the teacher creates an environment of scientific inquiry. Normalizing mistakes helps students accept and reflect on mistakes as the natural path for learning. Embody the message: all therapists make mistakes—including you (Casement, 1992). Our task is not to avoid mistakes but to learn from them.

As a fellow mistake-maker, model humility. Teachers can forget their struggles as beginners. Identify with the struggles of beginning therapists. Share your mistakes, confusion, and blind spots so that students will see these learning experiences as inevitable. "If my teacher had these struggles, worked hard, and succeeded, so can I."

Table 4.2 How to create a culture of mutual compassion for learning

Remind the group of the task. We are here to create a culture of mutual compassion for one another as fellow "mistake-makers."
Welcome all student responses.
Normalize making mistakes.
Remind students that all therapists make mistakes at all stages of their careers.
Mistakes are essential for learning.
Mistakes are opportunities to learn.
Our task is not to avoid mistakes but to learn from them. We are lifelong learners.

In the following example, metacognitive questions model how to treat mistakes as learning opportunities. A student reported feeling stuck with a passive patient. The teacher suggested that the student play the therapist. Then she, the teacher, would play the patient to learn why the therapy was stuck.

Student:	Give me the problem you would like me to help you with.
Teacher as patient:	I'll give you anything you want. I'm so glad to know therapy will be driven by your desire and not mine.
Student:	[*Surprised.*]
Teacher:	What are you learning? [*Metacognitive question to help the student reflect on what she is learning.*]
Student:	I hadn't realized I was asking the patient to give me something.
Teacher:	What impact might that have on your patient? [*Inviting the student to see how her intervention created the misalliance, keeping the therapy stuck.*]
Student:	He would feel like I am making demands on him. [*pause*] That's what he says about his girlfriend too. [*She is beginning to see how she is enacting the transference.*]
Teacher:	How might you revise your invitation, so that you don't step into the shoes of the demanding girlfriend?
Student:	What is the problem you would like me to help you with?
Teacher:	Right. So what was keeping this therapy stuck, do you think? [*A metacognitive question helps her see how her enactment supported the patient's passive transference. And that kept the therapy stuck.*]
Student:	If he thinks therapy is driven by my desire, it won't be driven by his desire. He'll go along with me like he does with his girlfriend.

Table 4.3 Metacognitive questions to help students think about a role-play

What are you learning?
What impact might that have on your patient?
How might you change your invitation to avoid stepping into the shoes of the demanding girlfriend?
What was keeping this therapy stuck, do you think?

The student knew she was stuck but not why. Everyone can see when a serve lands out of the tennis court. However, therapy mistakes are usually invisible. The student's problem became visible once she enacted it through role-play and experienced it. Her experience motivated her to find a new solution. Then the teacher's metacognitive questions helped her learn to think clinically.

Through these metacognitive questions, she can think about her approach. She can reflect on the impact of her actions on the patient. She can revise her interventions accordingly. And she can think about how her enactment kept the therapy stuck. She reached a new level of understanding and clinical thinking.

The metacognitive questions also taught the student a new form of causality. The patient was not keeping the therapy stuck. Instead, the student and patient both kept the therapy stuck. Thus, the student learned about cyclical causality (Grotzer & Mittelfehldt, 2012).

Students' mistakes are opportunities to teach clinical thinking. Metacognitive questions invite students to think about the patient's responses. Then, their answers can change their thinking. Sample metacognitive questions include:

- What can we learn from the patient's response?
- What is the patient's response teaching us?
- What supervision did the patient offer us?
- How does the patient's feedback change your hypothesis?
- And with that new hypothesis, how might you change your intervention?

A mistake provides students with an opportunity to take their thinking further. They can understand the patient more deeply and intervene more effectively. Thus, the teacher accepts mistakes as opportunities to teach, not judge. Judging is not teaching.

Students may fear criticism if they cannot answer a question. But the student's inability is not a problem; it's an opportunity. Ask yourself, "What does she not see that leads to this misunderstanding? What questions can I ask so that she can see that?"

Metacognizing about Feelings in the Learning Process

Since making mistakes is painful, normalize how struggling to learn triggers feelings. Then, students can reflect on their experiences of changing while learning.

For instance, invite students to reflect on their feelings and experiences in class.

- How are you feeling about this task, and how does that affect your learning?
- How does it feel to make mistakes together in front of one another?
- How does it feel not to understand something here when you wish you did?
- How does it feel when learning that this is harder than you thought it would be?
- When you struggle to learn this new skill, how do these feelings affect your learning?
- If you accepted it is difficult but possible to learn skills with hard work, how would that affect your learning?
- What feelings come up when you share your work in front of each other?
- It takes emotional courage to face anxiety when learning something new. What are you learning about your emotional courage?

Metacognitive questions help students reflect on their feelings while learning (metacognitive experiences). When students think about their struggles while learning, they integrate deep learning (Bion, 1965).

Transformative learning is never risk-free. "[T]o suggest that education can and should be risk-free ... is a misrepresentation of what education is about" (Biesta, 2006, pp. 25–26). It misrepresents life. So, we co-create a culture of compassion where students can take the risk of learning and evolving.

Principle: Ideally, we embody what we teach. Otherwise, what we do will conflict with what we teach, and students will do what we do, not what we teach.

Welcome mistakes as a form of collaboration.

Student: I made a mistake.
Teacher: Great that you saw that. Thank you for showing me where I can help you. You are helping me be a better teacher.

Students' errors supervise the teacher: "Help me here." There is no such thing as a stupid question. Questions reveal what the student has not been taught or has not integrated. Assess answers to find out what the student is not learning or integrating. Students' answers show where to focus the teaching. "Dumb" questions do not reflect on the student. They reveal what our teaching has failed to help him learn.

The narcissistic instructor misuses mistakes to judge the student, shaming her for needing help. Fifty percent of therapists have had harmful supervision (Ellis, Berger, & Siembor, 2013; Epstein, 1986). So be explicit about the learning environment you hope to co-create with them.

Beginning students may assume teachers have "the" answers. Instead, we have strategies for testing hypotheses we will refine or discard. Model the humility of clinical thinking: we admit when our thinking is off, revise it, and try again.

Teacher: That is a great question. Do you know why? I don't have an answer to it. So let's start with the facts and see what questions to ask to discover the answer.

Teacher: Given what we have heard in this session, do we know why the patient is hesitant? No, we don't. And we can't. All we know is she hesitates. There must be a good reason she is reluctant, but we don't know what it is. We could make stuff up, but we would be speculating instead of thinking. So, let's keep listening to the patient's responses and see what she can teach us. Then, we can put more pieces together to develop a more nuanced picture of her.

Model "not knowing" as normal when coming to know any person. Also, remind students you are not the supervisor. You are merely helping students listen to the true supervisor: the patient.

Even when we co-create a culture of compassion, anxiety can still rise in students. So, let's go to the next step: assessing and regulating anxiety in students.

Assessing and Regulating Anxiety in a Learning Group

When questions trigger students' anxiety, we can regulate it and return to the learning task.

Student: [*Racing speech, indicating anxiety is too high.*] This is all so confusing. I'm afraid I'm not going to be able to do it.

Teacher: [*Speaking slowly to calm the student. Cognizing to help the student begin to intellectualize.*] Thanks for letting me know. So, let's summarize what we have learned so far today. We have learned that when a patient shares a problem, he depends upon you. And depending may trigger anxiety in him. To reduce his anxiety, he may use defenses to avoid declaring a problem. As we replay the video segment, let's see what defenses he uses.

Regulate anxiety through your calm voice while intellectualizing about the learning problem. Once the student's anxiety drops, return to the educational task of assessing the patient's responses.

When questions are off the topic, answer the question briefly. Then, connect it to the educational focus and return to the task. In the following example, the instructor is teaching the defense of intellectualization.

Jim: How is this related to transference resistance? [*He asks an important question, but it takes us off the educational focus.*]
Teacher: Excellent question! That is a way of relating that has a defensive function [*Brief answer to the question. Then, pivot back to the educational focus.*] Coming back to intellectualization, who can offer an example of that defense?

If you ignore a student's question, anger will build up in the student, leading him to tune out. A brief answer will allow the student to feel heard while you return to the educational focus. If distracting questions continue, the group's anxiety may be too high.

As the psychotherapy field moves toward a more evidence-based approach to training (Haggerty & Hilsenroth, 2011; Kernberg, 2016), we use videotape more in teaching and supervision. However, supervising videotaped work triggers more anxiety in students (Topor et al., 2017). Why? Students cannot hide their mistakes. Thus, identify, normalize, and regulate students' anxiety so they learn to regulate it while revealing their work.

Use a video for active learning, not passive watching. Otherwise, students will learn to watch, not to think. When using videotape for teaching or supervision, stop after each response from the patient. Invite the class to assess the patient's response. Stopping frequently keeps the group's anxiety from rising too quickly. Ask the group to analyze each patient response and propose an intervention. Then, they will learn how clinical thinking leads to effective interventions.

Monitor and regulate the class's anxiety by going slowly. If necessary, intellectualize about the patient's response to regulate their anxiety. Keep the group on task. Watch a few seconds of the video. Next, invite them to analyze the patient's response and propose an intervention. Then repeat. When you maintain an effective educational focus in class or supervision, you model for them how to maintain a therapeutic focus with patients.

When students speculate, block speculation by asking for evidence from the patient. For instance, students may engage in egocentric thinking, believing that their feelings make a hypothesis true. However, a feeling from the therapist is not evidence from the patient.

Teacher: Yes, and your feeling is from you. What evidence do we have from the patient to support your hypothesis?

When you block speculation (anti-task behavior), you encourage clinical thinking (the task). Keep the group on task: analyzing the patient's responses to intervention.

Or the video may show the teacher exploring painful issues or feelings that the students usually avoid. As a result, the class's anxiety may spike, leading them to avoid the learning task by asking off-topic questions, withdrawing, or speculating about the patient. You can regulate the group's anxiety directly. Or you can provide more structure. Inviting the class to analyze each response from the patient before going to the next one prevents anxiety from rising too high. And it keeps students on the task of analyzing patient responses.

If the teacher believes the students are not "getting it," she may not be "getting" their anxiety. For instance, once, I presented a videotape of my work at a conference. Five minutes into the video, a student raised her hand and said, "I think this patient has lost his relationship with God." We had no evidence for that thought. Unable to tolerate her rising anxiety, the student projected onto the patient. Now, I knew she was the most anxious person in the group. If I could address her projection and anxiety, I could regulate the group's anxiety, too. I responded in the following fashion:

Teacher: Thank you for your idea. Is there any evidence for your hypothesis?

Student: Not yet.

Teacher: Okay. So, let's watch the videotape to see if the patient's responses confirm or disconfirm your hypothesis.

During the presentation, I kept inviting her to assess whether the patient's responses confirmed her hypothesis. Since I accepted her idea as a hypothesis to test, she felt accepted. And after she repeatedly saw that the patient's responses did not confirm her hypothesis, she could change it.

When the group analyzes a video, their answers allow the teacher to assess their anxiety. Does a class member suddenly have acute difficulty thinking? Or does she become quite confused? If so, is she getting too anxious? The most anxious student is the canary in the mine, who lets us know when anxiety is too high for the group. Sometimes, regulating the student regulates the group as well.

Teacher: When we have trouble thinking, it can be a sign of anxiety. Are you aware of feeling anxious as we cover this topic?

Student: Yes.

Teacher: Shall we help you with this anxiety so you can feel more comfortable?

Student: Okay.

Teacher: Where do you notice feeling this anxiety? [*The teacher helps the student identify and regulate her anxiety.*]

Student: In my stomach, like I'm sick to my stomach. [*Anxiety in the smooth muscles.*]

Teacher: Good to know. That's a high level of anxiety. So, something about our discussion of the patient's denial triggered some anxiety. And then the anxiety went to your gut. Does that fit your experience? [*The teacher intellectualizes about the process causing the student's anxiety to help regulate it.*]

Student: Yes. I think it reminded me of something in my family. [*The student can intellectualize, which is a good sign. And she sees the link that triggered her anxiety. The teacher will not explore the link because that is the task of therapy, not supervision. He regulates the student's anxiety so that she can return to the educational task.*]

Teacher: That makes sense. So, when we discussed the patient's denial, that stirred up something about your family. And that triggered some anxiety in your stomach. It's not a surprise that talking about emotional difficulties in patients will remind us of family issues. How is your anxiety now? [*The teacher intellectualizes about the process causing the student's anxiety to help regulate it. Plus, he normalizes the process: talking about patients' emotions will stir up our emotions and anxiety.*]

Student: It's okay now. [*Anxiety is regulated.*]

Teacher: Okay. Shall we come back to the question we were looking at before? [*With the student's anxiety regulated, the teacher returns to the educational task.*]

There are several ways to help the group with the anxiety aroused by showing videos of their work.

1 Normalize anxiety as an understandable reaction to revealing our work on video.
2 Remind the group that facing what makes us anxious helps us grow as therapists.
3 Share how anxious you were when you first showed your videotapes in supervision.
4 If a student remains anxious, ask her where she feels anxiety in her body. Then, ask about any thoughts about the class that make her uncomfortable. Once you have addressed her concerns, her anxiety will drop. Then, the class can resume its task: analyzing patient responses on the video.

How to Avoid Unnecessary Anxiety Triggers

Although learning skills triggers anxiety, teachers can avoid some anxiety triggers. For example, if you rarely ask questions, students will become anxious when you do. However, if you ask questions in every class, they will no longer evoke anxiety. If a teacher makes a big deal out of mistakes, students will fear judgment. Help students see errors as a natural part of our learning curve. The student's anxiety will rise if she has little time to think when asked a question. But, if you give her a few seconds, her struggle will help her see what she needs to learn.

> *Principle*: Allow students to struggle, so they experience where they need to direct their learning. They will also learn how hard work leads to mastery.

If teachers treat repetition as an inconvenience, students will fear asking questions. However, if teachers treat repetition as a natural part of learning complex concepts and skills, students will not fear asking questions. Students' questions help the teacher assess what students do not understand and why. They reveal the learning problem or problem about learning to focus on. If a student asks a question again, assess the new learning need. Rather than assume the student was not listening, listen more carefully.

- What decision tree questions could I ask to discover the learning problem that prevents her from integrating this new information?
- What feedback-driven metacognitive questions could I ask to assess what she is and is not integrating?
- What can I help her integrate so that her understanding changes?

Sometimes, the student does not change. If so, welcome that supervision from the student. Then, you and she can explore how to shift the teaching and supervision so that her work can change.

Teacher: How does this new information change your old knowledge?
Student: It hasn't. My knowledge about this is the same.
Teacher: Thanks for letting me know! When knowledge doesn't change, our work doesn't change. So let's see if we can help your knowledge change, so your work with the patient will change, too.

> *Principle*: All student responses offer conscious and unconscious supervision to the teacher, telling her where students need help.

Common Responses to the Anxiety of Learning

Shame: Always normalize errors. While raising my hands, I ask students, "How many of you make mistakes with patients?" Everyone raises their hands and smiles. Then I respond, "Thank heavens, I'm not the only one." Normalize mistakes to shift a shame-focused group to a learning group. Students who have been shamed for making mistakes expect to be shamed. Deactivate this projection.

Idealization: Students often long for an ideal teacher who knows everything. "If my teacher knows everything, I could too and never make mistakes." But everyone makes mistakes. No therapist succeeds 100% of the time. Remind them of that fact. Otherwise, students will idealize the teacher or method and devalue themselves. Then, they become depressed, unable to meet an unrealistic ideal. Or they become angry with an idealized teacher or model. Deactivate idealization so that real learning can begin.

Magic: Therapy is hard work. No wonder students may wish for an intervention that causes immediate and permanent change. For example, students may ask, "Does this model help with everything?" Implicitly, they ask, "Is your model magic?"

Teacher: Nothing is helpful with everything. Only magic does that. But the research shows this model is quite beneficial for many conditions. I can't offer you magic, but I can help you become more competent.

Always teach a model as a valuable tool for exploration, not a magical answer. Unfortunately, some teachers imply that their model is ideal and devalue other models. They teach devaluation instead of clinical thinking. And the class becomes a cult (Abbass, 2004; Kernberg, 2016).

We cannot teach omnipotence, only mere competence. Always deactivate the fantasy of omnipotence.

Student: Do you ever make mistakes?
Teacher: All the time. It's how I learn from patients. For instance, let me tell you about my biggest mistake as a therapist. [*Deactivate idealization so that a realistic teaching relationship can develop.*]

Therapy is complex and challenging. Students may wish for a formula, method, or idealized teacher. Instead, prepare students for the hard work of being lifelong learners.

Domination/submission: Some students ask, "Am I supposed to believe this?" The student may be enacting his history. Perhaps he had to parrot a teacher's thoughts rather than develop his own. If he perceives you as a tyrant, he will oppose what you teach.

Teacher: Of course not. In religious cults, people believe in fixed doctrines. In therapy, we test hypotheses so our theory can evolve. When we intervene, we assess the patient's response to our intervention. Did the patient's response validate our hypothesis? If so, great. If not, great. We can try to form a better one and keep testing it until we are on the right track. So please do not believe anything I say here. When I hear your cases, I can only offer hypotheses for you to test. The patients will tell us which hypotheses are validated. Our task is to listen to patients, our true supervisors and teachers.

A common test for the teacher takes this form:

Student: Would it be okay to intervene this way? [*Do I have to submit to you and say what you tell me?*]

Teacher: I don't know if that intervention would be okay. Do you know why?

Student: No.

Teacher: We haven't heard the patient's response to the intervention yet. The patient's response determines whether the intervention would be helpful. Shall we listen to the patient's response so that she can teach us? [*Differentiate submission to a teacher from clinical thinking based on scientific method. The patient, not the teacher, determines whether an intervention worked.*]

Student: Yes.

Teacher: In a sense, I'm not the teacher. I'm only here to help you learn to listen to the real teacher: the patient. [*Clarify the educational task: learning to learn from the patient.*]

Principle: Do not teach students to listen to you. Teach them to listen to the real teacher and supervisor: the patient.

This problem about learning can manifest in another form:

Student: Do we have to say it this way? Would it be okay if I said, "I hear you think your wife has sexual issues. Could you say how that impacts your inner life?" [*The student turns to me rather than to the patient's responses. If I answered his question, the conflict would be between his hypothesis and mine. Instead, we can invite him to compare his hypothesis with the evidence, thereby teaching the scientific method.*]

Teacher:	Of course, you could start the session that way. [*Deactivating the projection that I want to control him.*] Shall we do a role-play and see how that intervention works?
Student:	Okay. I hear you think your wife has sexual issues. Could you say how that impacts your inner life?
Teacher as patient:	Her sexual issues affect my inner life a lot. [*Create an experience to help the student experience the problem in his intervention.*]
Student:	But how is it impacting your inner life?
Teacher as patient:	I'm so frustrated sexually, and it hurts me. Could you help me convince her to have more sex? [*Create an experience to help the student experience the problem in his intervention.*]
Student:	I'm not getting anywhere.
Teacher:	What defenses is the patient using that prevent *him* from getting anywhere? [*Inviting the student to think clinically about the patient's responses.*]
Student:	He blames his wife for his problems. And now it's as if he is saying he doesn't belong in therapy, his wife does.
Teacher:	Exactly. So let's go back to your invitation. You asked how his wife's sexual issues impact his inner life. Would that invite him to describe his problem or invite him to focus on his wife as the problem? [*Helping the student evaluate the effect of his intervention.*]
Student:	Got it. I invited him to talk about how his wife's problems were causing his problems. [*Now, the student can think about his intervention and its effect.*]
Teacher:	So how could you block his defense of blaming his wife by reminding him she is not here and invite him to tell you about his problem he wants help with?
Student:	Since your wife is not here, I can't help her. So what is the problem you would like me to help you with?

The student learns that we assess an intervention based on the patient's response. Through role-play, he experiences an intervention's effect. Then he can change his thinking and intervention. Rather than rely on the teacher's approval, he listens to the patient's response.

Another example of learning through submission took this form:

Student: Did I do it right? [*Problem about learning: the student learns through submission.*]

Teacher: I can't know because I'm not your patient. Let's listen to the patient's response to your intervention to see if it validates your hypothesis. [*Block learning by submission to the teacher. Then encourage the student to learn from the patient.*]

Do not ask students to give up their ideas. Instead, invite them to compare their ideas with data from the patient. In class, treat every idea as acceptable for testing. If students think a teacher wants them to believe her mind rather than develop their own, she will receive submission or opposition. Neither attitude would foster learning.

Principle: The student should never submit to the teacher. Our hypotheses submit to the evidence from the patient.

Help the student assess whether the patient's response fits his hypothesis. Then, the student learns that he is not required to believe a teacher or a theory. Instead, he learns to use patients' responses to change his thinking and interventions. When the teacher is open to students' hypotheses, students learn to be open to their patients' responses.

Treat students' beliefs and assumptions as hypotheses to test in the spirit of scientific inquiry. Then, they can improve their thinking about and understanding of patients. However, learning requires students to tolerate frustration when they make mistakes.

Manage Frustration to Manage Projection in the Group

Making mistakes in class is frustrating. If students end an exercise with a mistake, they become demoralized. They may judge themselves and assume the teacher does, too. Manage frustration in students by promoting mastery. For instance, repeat deliberate practice exercises until they master them. Then, they will no longer judge themselves or imagine the teacher does. Success will excite them to learn more.

Manage time to reduce frustration. If students have trouble with a new concept, ask a question, then pause a few seconds before calling on a student. Give the class more time to think to find a better answer. As they get better at thinking with the new concept, ask questions more quickly in cold calls. If offering more time does not help them, consider breaking your question down into parts so they can tackle it bit by bit.

Students can also become frustrated if they imagine you are judging or criticizing them. Block the projection of judgment and encourage self-compassion.

Example of projection onto the teacher

Student: I feel like you're criticizing me.

Teacher: Thanks for letting me know. I wasn't talking about you at all. I was talking about the hypothesis, which is a plausible one. If the hypothesis is off, that isn't a criticism of you. It is just a sign that the hypothesis needs revision. How does this focus on the hypothesis change your understanding of what we are paying attention to?

Student: I thought you were criticizing me. But I see now that you are focusing on the hypothesis.

Teacher: Yes. The focus isn't on you but on the hypothesis. Shall we turn our attention to the hypothesis now? And then, let's see if the patient's responses validate it.

When a teacher points out problems in a student's thinking, he may think she criticized him. Remind him that you were not talking about him but his hypothesis. Help the student differentiate himself from his thoughts so he can think about them. Calling his thoughts a "hypothesis" helps him observe rather than identify with them. As a result, he can compare his thoughts to the patient's responses.

In the following vignette, a student shows a video of a patient shaking in her chair who fears the therapist will criticize her. Then, the patient says she wants to get up and leave the session. The teacher helps the student engage in metacognition.

Teacher: You're right. She is very anxious. Why do you suppose she is so anxious right now? [*What does the student see and not see? Assessing her learning need.*]

Student: She said she was afraid I would criticize her. [*She sees the statement but not its implications.*]

Teacher: And is this merely an idea she has about you, or does she believe it? [*Can the student see that the patient has temporarily lost her reality testing?*]

Student: I hadn't thought about it like that. [*She reveals part of her learning need.*]

Teacher: If you think about it this way, is this merely an idea, or does she believe it?

Student: She believes it.

Teacher: So, when she believes this idea, is she relating to you, or is she interacting with a projection? [*Can the student think about the impact of the projection on the relationship?*]

Student: Uh. Relating to a projection.

Teacher: So if she left your office, would she be leaving you or trying to leave a projection back in the office? [*Can the student think about the relationship between acting out and the projection?*]

Student: Wow! I never thought about why she was thinking about leaving.

Teacher: What effect might this projection have on her anxiety? [*Can the student see the impact that projection would have on the patient's anxiety?*]

Student: If she believes I would criticize her, her anxiety will get worse. [*Now the student can see causality.*]

Teacher: So, if projection makes her anxiety worse, how might we reduce her anxiety? [*Using the concept of causality, can she think of the intervention to use?*]

Student: Make projection less?

Teacher: Exactly. So, let's look at some interventions to deactivate her projection, so she could connect to you rather than run away from a projection. [*The instructor teaches the skills the student doesn't have.*]

This student could not figure out what the problem was. So, the teacher asked a series of decision tree questions to discern her learning need. Then he could help her see what she hadn't seen. Once she saw the projection, she understood the patient's urge to leave. Then, she could deactivate the projection to restore the therapeutic alliance.

Encouraging Hard Work When Learning Is Hard

All learning requires us to work slightly beyond our skill level. Dynamic teaching stretches us to do something new, unfamiliar, and uncomfortable. The student moves out of her comfort zone into the learning zone to grow (Vygotsky, 1978). Thus, we always convey our faith in her ability to learn and grow. When she reaches beyond her current level of understanding, she will be more active and more likely to integrate new concepts. As soon as she learns one skill, we move to a harder one; the window of learning keeps moving forward.

Nevertheless, moving from the comfort zone into the learning zone causes distress. No wonder students can prefer ineffective training such as attending conferences. In contrast, supervision of videotapes and skill-building (Baddeley & Longman, 1978) causes anxiety.

Students need support. Do not praise them for being smart, a matter of genetic luck. Instead, praise them for working hard in the face of difficulty. Two factors drive teaching success: good teachers encourage students to work hard, and students feel motivated by their connection to the teacher

(Lemov, 2021). Remind students that you offer feedback because you believe in their potential. Then, they can use criticism constructively (Aguilar, Walton, & Wieman, 2014; Yeager et al., 2013). Here are some examples of feedback that help students during deliberate practice in class or supervision.

- It was hard for me, too. That's why I know you can do it if you practice like I did.
- Yes, it is hard. Shall we help you develop those skills?
- As you keep practicing, your skill will increase. Shall we practice more so you can master it?
- Keep going when you make mistakes. Mistakes reveal your weak spot so you can get stronger. Every therapist has had to go through struggles like you. It's how you can become an expert. Let's keep at it until you master it.

Student: Do we have to do these exercises?
Teacher: Of course not. But then you will get stuck when these problems come up with your patients. Shall we practice them now, so you won't get stuck later?
Student: But this is so hard!
Teacher: Yes, that's why it is hard with your patients, too. Shall we practice it now so it will be easier to help them?

Learning skills in class creates "desirable difficulties" (Bjork, 1994), the ones that students will have with patients. We want them to experience the difficulties in class they will encounter in the clinic. For instance, if a student works with patients who do not trust her, we help her learn how to deactivate projections that create distrust. Difficulties arise in clinical work. Thus, experiencing and mastering those difficulties in supervision is desirable.

While desirable difficulties do not feel good, they are good to have. We help students become comfortable with discomfort because discomfort arises in therapy. Make the challenges of a class match those in the clinic. Otherwise, the class will not prepare students for the real world and, thus, will not engage them.

Metacognitive Self-Regulation Strategies

Integrating new information makes old knowledge dissolve. Yet positive disintegration triggers anxiety, which can be dysregulating. Therefore, we can help the student by offering metacognitive self-regulation strategies. The following checklist can help students organize their understanding of the therapeutic task. Then, they can bear the dysregulation of positive disintegration.

Table 4.4 A checklist of metacognitive questions for self-regulation

Planning

1. What are the patient's goals for therapy?
2. What therapeutic task will help the patient achieve that goal?
3. What information would help you assess the patient, and what strategies could you use to get that information?

Monitoring

1. How do you understand what you are doing?
2. How does the therapeutic task make sense to the patient and you?
3. Is the patient reaching her goals?
4. What changes in approach are you considering?

Evaluating

1. To what extent has the patient reached her goals?
2. What worked?
3. What didn't work?
4. What will you do differently next time?

Source: Adapted from Schraw, 1998.

Metacognitive Regulation of Positive Disintegration

A student was struggling to understand the concept of conflict. She knew she was confused but could not describe what was confusing her. So I suggested that she think about it and write down what she found confusing about conflict in preparation for the next class. The next day she described what she had learned.

Student: I figured out my problem. I am trying to integrate this with the previous kinds of therapy I learned. And I couldn't mash them together.

Teacher: That makes sense. You can never mash two models of therapy together. Anything new you learn always contradicts something you know. So, the problem is that old knowledge disintegrates a bit to integrate new information.

Student: I couldn't do it. And I didn't know why. And then, at the end of our training yesterday, I really felt despair.

Teacher: Sure, because old knowledge despairs, knowing it disintegrates while integrating new information. How does that change your understanding of what happens when you take in new information?

Student: Well, I'm still alive.

Teacher: That's a profound insight! You see, when old knowledge integrates new knowledge, it is threatened. "I'm dying. I'm dying." And when old knowledge dies, we can feel like we are dying too.

But only an old way of thinking is dying, and a new integrated form of thinking is born. So, how does your understanding change when you see old knowledge was dying and not you?

Student: I feel excited!

Changing an idea, assumption, or belief changes the student's self-state. And on an unconscious level, a change of self-state equals death. All deep learning is experienced unconsciously as the death of oneself. No wonder students can feel so threatened by the changes occurring during psychotherapy training (Bion, 1962). Thus, addressing the fear of dying through learning can reduce the resistance to change.

Metacognitive questions can help students observe and reflect on their feelings of positive disintegration. Then, they can regulate themselves during the dysregulation caused by learning. For example, the following metacognitive questions can help students regulate themselves while learning:

- Of the new information you learned today, what changed your old knowledge the most?
- What new information are you having the most difficulty integrating? What is making it difficult to integrate?
- What feelings does integrating this new information stir up?
- When feelings come up, how do they affect your learning? What new information does your old knowledge want to avoid?
- When we learn, old knowledge disintegrates, letting new knowledge come in. What information has felt most threatening to your prior knowledge?
- What have you learned about the difficulty old knowledge has when taking in new information?
- Are you the knowledge you learned in the past? Or is knowledge a tool you use for thinking? How does that change your perspective on knowledge?
- Are you a theory (e.g., CBT)? Or is a theory a tool you use for thinking? How does that change your perspective on yourself, a thinker who uses theories as tools for thinking?
- Are you a listening approach (reflection)? Or is reflection just one way you can listen? How does that change your perspective as a therapist who chooses which listening strategies to use?
- When this learning process makes you anxious, are you in danger? Or is an old way of thinking in danger of changing? How does this change your perspective on the risk of using new concepts to think about patients?

Why Anxiety Rises in Contemporary Teaching

Listening to lectures and talking in class are easy. So doing therapy may appear easy, too (Jacoby & Kelley, 1987). Speedy answers may show how well students have memorized a fact. However, a correct answer on a test does not measure skills with patients. In fact, familiarity with a domain of knowledge makes us vulnerable to illusions of mastery (Reder, 1987, 1988; Reder & Ritter, 1992; Schwartz & Metcalfe, 1992).

Students and teachers show their skills in music, chess, or sports. However, psychotherapy teachers rarely show their work. When students do not see teachers' therapy skills, skill remains an abstract concept. They cannot assess their skill level without answering questions, analyzing videos, or doing skill-building exercises. Then, mistakes they do not make in class occur with patients instead.

Integrating research from the learning sciences, we use decision tree questions, skill-building exercises, role-plays, and video analyses. In an active, dialogical form of learning, students will make more mistakes and become more anxious. And positive disintegration becomes much more prominent.

Relational Pedagogy

We help students with the process of conceptual change through a relational pedagogy. In a relational form of pedagogy, we teach and then assess the student's responses to our teaching. Her responses supervise our subsequent interventions. What supervision does the student's answer give? Does she need help bearing anxiety or positive disintegration? Did she use a folk assumption? Did she offer a new learning problem? Is she revealing a problem about learning? What does her answer tell me about what she has trouble integrating? The student's conscious and unconscious supervision informs our interventions. Each student response supervises the teacher. Then, we revise our teaching/supervision strategy and intervene again, waiting for the next student response (the supervision of the teacher/supervisor).

When addressing positive disintegration, acknowledge students' fear of change. Then, pay attention to their anxiety to build trust in the teaching/ learning relationship (Bovill, 2020). Help them bear their anxiety while their old ways of knowing and relating dissolve. Then they can integrate new learning. Caring for their distress while they learn reveals how "teaching and learning are relational activities" (Werder et al., 2010, p. 38).

In a relational pedagogy, decision tree questions offer a form of dialogical reasoning. While the questions are structured, students' responses are unpredictable. They may reveal learning problems. For instance, what fact, concept, skill, or technique would help the student most today? Or their responses may expose problems about learning. For example, what habits or attitudes interfere with the student's learning (Ekstein & Wallerstein, 1972)? Then a genuine dialogue emerges. The teacher empathizes with the student's inevitable learning struggle. Through dialogue, the student learns a kind of interpersonal reasoning. She discovers how to communicate with a particular patient. She begins to understand how patients perceive her words. She also discovers how patients' responses can change her clinical thinking.

> *Principle*: Welcome supervision from the student, so that she will welcome supervision from the patient.

Every student's answer co-creates the ongoing conscious and unconscious dialogue of learning. Thus, the teacher understands all student responses as conscious and unconscious supervision. "The teacher is no longer the-one-who-teaches, but who is [herself] taught in dialogue with the students, who in turn while being taught also teach" (Freire, 2003, p. 63). Thus, teaching and supervision exemplify a relational epistemology (Ananda, Medin, & ojhleto, 2018; Thayer-Bacon, 1997).

> *Principle*: The teacher is not the "teller who knows all." She receives supervision from students' responses on how to teach. As a learner, she models for students how to receive supervision from their patients.

Teaching does not consist of the monological delivery of a finite set of facts to a student. Instead, teaching is a dialogical process. Together, the teacher and student examine patient responses and create new knowledge. The teacher assesses the student's learning need, intervenes, and assesses the student's responses. This process parallels how the student assesses the patient's need, intervenes, and assesses the patient's responses.

In this constructivist pedagogy (Kafai, 2022), students build their understanding of psychotherapy by doing the skills in class or supervision that they will need with patients. The student is no longer a passive listener. The teacher provides opportunities for learning by doing. Learning becomes "a process of active construction" where the student can "own the sense-making process" that takes place (Grotzer & Mittelfehldt, 2012, p. 95; Gunstone, 1991).

Summary

Integrating new information causes old knowledge to disintegrate. This inevitable positive disintegration causes anxiety in the learner. Normalize and regulate it so that the student can integrate new information and change. Now, we can shift to how we teach new psychological concepts and thinking skills—declarative knowledge.

Questions for Teachers and Supervisors to Ask about Students

- What emotions are students having during the learning process?
- What emotional reactions interfere with students' learning?
- What reactions from a supervisee or class let you know their anxiety has become too high?
- What misconceptions about the class emerge with an increase in anxiety?
- What are you learning from the students' responses to your attempts to foster anxiety regulation?

References

Abbass, A. (2004). Idealization and devaluation as barriers to psychotherapy learning. *Ad Hoc Bulletin of Short-Term Dynamic Psychotherapy, 8*(3), 46–55.

Aguilar, L., Walton, G., & Wieman, C. (2014). Psychological insights for improved physics teaching. *Physics Today, 67,* 43–49.

Alonso, A., & Rutan, S. (1988). Shame and guilt in supervision. *Psychotherapy Theory, Research, and Practice, 25*(4), 576–581. https://doi.org/10.1037/h0085384

Ananda, M., Medin, D., & ojlehto, b. (2018). Conceptual change, relationship, and cultural epistemologies. In T. Amin & O. Levrini (Eds.), *Converging perspectives on conceptual change: Mapping the emerging paradigm in the learning sciences* (pp. 43–50). New York: Routledge.

Arkowitz, S. (2001). Perfectionism in the supervisee. In S. Gill (Ed.), *The supervisory alliance: Facilitating the supervisee's learning experience* (pp. 3–66). Northvale, N.J.: Jason Aronson.

Baddeley, A., & Longman, D. (1978). The influence of length and frequency of training session on the rate of learning to type. *Ergonomics, 21,* 627–635.

Biesta, G. (2006). *Beyond learning: Democratic education for a human future.* London: Paradigm Publishers.

Bion, W. R. (1962). *Learning from experience.* London: William Heinemann.

Bion, W. R. (1965). *Transformations: Change from learning to growth.* London: Heinemann.

Bjork, R. A. (1994). Memory and metamemory considerations in the training of human beings. In J. Metcalfe & A. Shimamura (Eds.), *Metacognition: Knowing about knowing* (pp. 185–205). Cambridge, Mass.: MIT Press.

Boser, U. (2017). *Learn better: Mastering the skills for success in life, business, and school, or How to become an expert in just about anything.* New York: Rodale Books.

Bovill, C. (2020). *Co-creating learning and teaching: Towards relational pedagogy in higher education.* St. Albans, UK: Critical Publishing.

Casement, P. (1992). *Learning from the patient.* New York: Guilford Press.

Dabrowski, K. (2017). *Positive disintegration.* Anna Maria, Fla.: Maurice Bassett.

Ekstein, R., & Wallerstein, R. (1972). *The teaching and learning of psychotherapy.* New York: International Universities Press.

Ellis, M., Berger, L., & Siembor, M. (2013). Inadequate and harmful clinical supervision: Testing a revised framework and assessing occurrence. *The Counseling Psychologist, 42*(4), 434–472.

Epstein, L. (1986). Collusive selective inattention to the negative impact of the supervisory interaction. *Contemporary Psychoanalysis, 22*(3), 389–409.

Freire, P. (2003). From pedagogy of the oppressed. In A. Darder, M. Baltodano, & R. Torres (Eds.), *The critical pedagogy reader.* New York: Routledge.

Grotzer, T., & Mittelfehldt, S. (2012). The role of metacognition in students' understanding and transfer of explanatory structures in science. In A. Zohar & Y. Dori (Eds.), *Metacognition in science education: Trends in current research* (pp. 79–99). New York: Springer.

Gunstone, R. F. (1991). Reconstructing theory from practical experience. In B. E. Woolnough (Ed.), *Practical science* (pp. 67–77). Milton Keynes, UK: Open University Press.

Haggerty, G., & Hilsenroth, M. J. (2011). The use of video in psychotherapy supervision. *British Journal of Psychotherapy, 27*(2), 193–210.

Hahn, W. (2001). The experience of shame in psychotherapy supervision. *Psychotherapy Theory, Research, and Practice, 38*(3), 272–282.

Jacoby, L., & Kelley, C. (1987). Unconscious influences of memory for a prior event. *Personality and Social Psychology Bulletin, 13*, 314–336.

Kafai, Y. (2022). Constructionism. In R. Sawyer (Ed.), *The Cambridge handbook of the learning sciences* (pp. 35–46). Cambridge, UK: Cambridge University Press.

Kernberg, O. (2016). *Psychoanalytic education at the crossroads: Reformation, change and the future of psychoanalytic training.* New York: Routledge.

Lemov, D. (2021). *Teach like a champion 3.0.* New York: Jossey-Bass.

Metcalfe, J., & Shimamura, J. (Eds.). (1994). *Metacognition: Knowing about knowing.* Cambridge, Mass.: MIT Press.

Owens, D., Sadler, T., Barlow, A., & Smith-Walters, C. (2020). Student motivation from and resistance to active learning rooted in essential science practices. *Research in Science Education, 50*, 253–277.

Reder, L. (1987). Strategy selection in question answering. *Cognitive Psychology, 19*, 90–138.

Reder, L., & Ritter, F. (1992). What determines initial feeling of knowing? Familiarity with question terms, not with the answer. *Journal of Experimental Psychology: Learning, Memory, and Cognition, 18*, 435–452.

Reder, L. M. (1988). Strategic control of retrieval strategies. In G. H. Bower (Ed.), *The psychology of learning and motivation: Advances in research and theory, Vol. 22* (pp. 227–259). Cambridge, Mass.: Academic Press.

Rumelhart, D., & Norman, D. (1978). Accretion, tuning and restructuring: Three modes of learning. In J. W. Cotton & R. Klatzky (Eds.), *Semantic factors in cognition* (pp. 37–53). Hillsdale, N.J.: Erlbaum.

Schraw, G. (1998). Promoting general metacognitive awareness. *Instructional Science, 26*, 113–125.

Schwartz, B., & Metcalfe, J. (1992). Cue familiarity but not target retrievability enhances feeling-of-knowing judgments. *Journal of Experimental Psychology: Learning, Memory, and Cognition, 18*, 1074–1083.

Talbot, N. (1995). Unearthing shame in the supervisory experience. *American Journal of Psychotherapy, 49*(3), 338–349. https://doi.org/10.1176/appi.psychotherapy.1995.49.3.338

Thayer-Bacon, B. (1997). The nurturing of a relational epistemology. *Educational Theory, 47*(2), 239–260.

Topor, D. R., AhnAllen, C. G., Mulligan, E. A., & Dickey, C. C. (2017). Using video recordings of psychotherapy sessions in supervision: Strategies to reduce learner anxiety. *Academic Psychiatry, 41*(1), 40–43.

Vygotsky, L. (1978). *Mind in society: The development of higher psychological processes*. Cambridge, Mass.: Harvard University Press.

Werder, C., Ware, L., Thomas, C., & Skogsburg, E. (2010). Students in parlor talk on teaching and learning. In C. Werder, & M. Otis (Eds.), *Engaging student voices in the study of teaching and learning* (pp. 16–31). Sterling, Va.: Stylus.

Yeager, D., Garcia, G., Bruztoski, P., Hessert, W., Purdie-Vaughns, V., Apfel, N., & Cohen, G. (2013). Breaking the cycle of mistrust: Wise interventions to provide critical feedback across the racial divide. *Journal of Experimental Psychology: General, 143*(2), 804–824.

Zohar, A., & Barzilai, S. (2015). Teaching higher order thinking in science education. In R. Wegeriff, & J. Kaufman (Eds.) *The Routledge international handbook of research on teaching thinking* (pp. 229–242). New York: Routledge.

Chapter 5

Declarative Knowledge: The Facts and Concepts We Use for Clinical Thinking

Jon Frederickson

Clinical Thinking: The Types of Knowledge

Most domains of expertise rely on four types of knowledge (Anderson & Krathwohl, 2001). Across disciplines, instructors teach:

1 *Declarative knowledge*: the facts and concepts of the field. Students learn to use a theory and its concepts as tools for clinical thinking.
2 *Procedural knowledge*: how to put theory into practice, translating clinical thinking into interventions.
3 *Conditional knowledge*: when, why, and with whom we use specific skills and interventions.
4 *Metacognitive knowledge*: what we learn by thinking about our thinking, our interventions, and patients' responses to them. We assess whether an intervention helped the patient. Then, patients' feedback can change our thinking and interventions. As a result, we can observe and control our learning (Schraw, 2006). And that process of changing our thinking turns students into lifelong learners (Anderson & Krathwohl, 2001). Metacognitive questions help students integrate declarative, procedural, and conditional knowledge.

Declarative knowledge (Factual knowledge): *what* we know. Students learn basic facts and concepts of psychotherapy (Bruner, 1961) to solve psychological problems. Yet, recalling a fact does not mean the student can use it for clinical thinking. An iPhone can record facts. However, only a student who can use them for clinical thinking knows them in practice. For instance, can she identify anxiety in a patient, think about its cause, and regulate it?

Declarative knowledge (Conceptual knowledge): the theory and concepts we use for clinical thinking. Concepts allow us to categorize facts. We use concepts like anxiety, defense, and conflict to see patterns we would not otherwise perceive. For example, a patient's trembling (fact) indicates

DOI: 10.4324/9781003488637-5

she suffers from anxiety (concept). Next, we can use the concept of conflict to understand what causes the patient's anxiety. She is angry with a husband who betrayed her. Anger triggers her anxiety. And to avoid it, she uses a defense—rationalizing his behavior. Thus, a concept (conflict) allows the student to see a pattern (feelings, anxiety, defense) in the patient's words and behaviors.

Procedural knowledge: *how* the therapist puts declarative knowledge into practice through listening, thinking, and intervention skills. Those skills can include:

- Establishing a therapeutic focus
- Anxiety identification and regulation
- Exploring feelings
- Defense identification
- Listening to latent content

Metacognitive knowledge: Thinking about our thinking and learning results in metacognitive knowledge. The student learns to think about the concepts she uses for clinical thinking. Then, she can analyze how her clinical thinking leads to interventions. Next, she can assess whether the patient's response confirms her hypothesis. Can she think about how new information from the patient changes her old knowledge? If so, she can change her hypotheses and interventions. She can grow because she is learning from the patient (Casement, 1992, 2019; Langs, 1989a, 1989b).

One might say declarative knowledge is *what* students know. Procedural knowledge is *how* they put it into practice. Conditional knowledge is *when* and *why* we use those concepts and skills. And metacognitive knowledge is what we learn when we think about our thinking, interventions, and patients' responses to our interventions.

First, students learn clinical facts and concepts. Next, they learn to use concepts to think clinically about facts. Then, students form hypotheses and test them through interventions. Finally, students can assess patient responses to improve their thinking and interventions. As a result, their understanding of the patient deepens (Hofmann & Hayes, 2021; Langs, 1989a, 1989b; Peterfreund, 2020; Raney, 1983; Rubovitz-Seitz, 2002).

Students often mistake facts they memorize for knowledge. For instance, "Aaron Beck developed the psychotherapy model known as cognitive therapy." But this is inert knowledge. It *does* nothing (Bransford, Brown, & Cocking, 2000). Instead, we teach students how to *use* concepts to *organize* clinical facts (e.g., what the patient says and does in session) into patterns that reveal what causes the patient's suffering. Through using concepts for clinical thinking, students *acquire* knowledge. This dynamic knowledge tells the student how and why to intervene. Once students have these

Table 5.1 The types of knowledge

Type of Knowledge	Definition
Declarative Knowledge	The facts and concepts we use to solve psychological problems through clinical thinking.
Procedural Knowledge	The skills we use and the steps we take to put theory into practice.
Conditional Knowledge	When, why, and with whom we use those concepts and skills.
Metacognitive Knowledge	The knowledge gained when we think about our thinking, interventions, and learning process.

thinking and intervention skills and see how they work together, they have deep knowledge.

All genuine therapy models use psychological concepts to engage in clinical thinking. The teaching principles apply to any model of therapy based on a comprehensive psychological theory, for example, cognitive/behavioral therapy, behavior therapy, or psychoanalysis.

The Goal of Teaching and Supervising

People may mistakenly regard the learning of content as the educational goal. But knowing the word "car" does not mean you can drive one. Likewise, a student may know the term "chain behavior analysis" but be unable to do that analysis in a session.

Defining a concept is superficial knowledge. Deep knowledge means that we know how to use it to intervene effectively. Thus, developing deep knowledge is the goal. Then we can plan how to help students become effective therapists (Zohar, 2012). Since thinking, listening, and intervention skills are explicit educational goals, let us turn to the teaching of declarative knowledge.

Retrieval: Teaching the Skill of Retrieving Key Facts and Concepts

In the "vessel" school of teaching, the lecturer pours information into the student's head. Then he hopes it stays there, like wine in a bottle. However, that's not how memory works. We forget most of what we learn unless we relearn it very soon and repeatedly (Japp, Muerre, & Dros, 2015). According to researcher Scott Freeman, giving a lecture is educational "malpractice" (Boser, 2017, p. 27). Why? As soon as we learn new information, we forget up to 50% the next day and 75% a week later. This predictable drop in memory is called the *forgetting curve* (Ebbinghaus, 1913/2014).

The forgetting curve does not result from an information processing problem. Forgetting always happens in learning (Roediger, Weinstein, & Agarwal, 2010). Thus, students' knowledge remains shallow after lectures and not functional in the real world (National Research Council, 2007; Wright & Boggs, 2002). After all, what a student forgets, she cannot use. In a meta-analysis of 225 studies (Freeman et al., 2014), the lecture format resulted in 50% more student failures than the active learning format. A similar result in a drug trial would terminate the study.

The best way to teach declarative knowledge is through retrieval, spacing, and interleaving (Dunlosky et al., 2013; Roediger, 2013). Repeatedly ask students to retrieve what they learned. Invite them to put new information into their words. And ask questions that have them practice applying that information so that new facts and skills become stored in long-term memory (Pashler et al., 2007). Retrieval shows effects that are up to 50% higher than from other forms of learning (Agarwal & Bain, 2019). Why? When students can retrieve knowledge, they can use it (Roediger, Weinstein, & Agarwal, 2010).

Students either retrieve knowledge or forget it.

Do not give a standard lecture. Instead, offer an engaged lecture. Here, the teacher often stops and asks students, "What did you just learn?" First, call on them randomly, so that everyone is accountable. Then ask other students to summarize what the previous student said. Then ask the first student if the second student accurately presented his point of view. When students put knowledge in their words, they are more likely to remember it (Lemov, 2021). Ask frequent retrieval questions to interrupt the forgetting curve.

Teachers often focus on getting information into students' heads. But telling is not teaching. Instead, focus on getting information *out* of students' heads. Rather than tell students what they have read, ask what they learned. The word "educate" derives from the Latin *educare*, meaning to bring forth knowledge from the student. Students often say, "I know we talked about it, but I couldn't remember it until after the session." When teachers tell facts and concepts, students do not retrieve them. And if they do not retrieve them in class, they will not be able to with patients.

As the student did not remember new information during the session, he could not use this knowledge. Remembering it after the session did him no good. This is why working on retrieval in class or supervision is so important. Then, he will retrieve this information when he needs it: in the next session.

Students learn a little when teachers tell them what to learn (the stage of encoding memory). But most learning occurs during retrieval when *students* describe what they have learned (Agarwal, Bain, & Chamberlain,

2012; Brown, Roedinger, & McDaniel, 2014). Retrieval boosts memory more than additional study (Landauer & Bjork, 1978). Of course, homework and critical reading are valuable. (See McGuire & McGuire, 2015, for metacognitive strategies for students studying their readings.) However, retrieval during an engaged lecture is essential for long-term learning.

Retrieval is up to 50% more effective a learning strategy than lecturing, re-reading, or taking notes (Roediger et al., 2010; Pashler et al., 2007).

When you ask students what they have learned, you put them on the spot. It raises their anxiety when they begin to forget. While retrieval is optimal for long-term memory, it is hard. Should learning be challenging for students? Researchers have found easy learning leads to short-term retention (Agarwal & Bain, 2019).

In contrast, slower strategies involving hard work result in long-term retention. Questions that cause students to struggle create a "desirable difficulty" (Bjork, 1994). Difficulties boost students' ability to retain and think about new information.

Every teacher has taught a concept that students do not remember later. Why? If students do not use a concept, it does not become usable, thus, memorable. We remember more of a story when we physically act it out (Scott, Harris, & Rothe, 2001). You do not become stronger by watching a weightlifter lift a barbell. Likewise, students do not become skillful thinkers by hearing a supervisor's thoughts. Students must practice skills repeatedly.

Principle: Students learn to think clinically by doing it. Are you doing the clinical thinking? Or are you asking questions, so that students do the clinical thinking?

Students do not store new information in long-term memory by recording it. Instead, information gets stored when students *integrate* it with their prior knowledge. Retrieval modifies a memory, making it easier to recall in the future (Bjork, 1975). Then, their new understanding becomes more holistic and personally meaningful.

Principle: Students remember new information according to what it means to them and how it links to what they know. Ask questions so that they make those links.

The teacher's primary responsibility is not to impart information but to help students integrate it. Thus, ask metacognitive questions:

1 How does this new information change your old knowledge?
2 What do you understand now that you did not understand before?
3 What do you see that you didn't see before?

These metacognitive questions help students link new information with old knowledge.

Principle: If students do not integrate new information, their understanding will not change nor their work. Therefore, ask metacognitive questions until change occurs.

While lecturing, a teacher cannot assess what students remember, integrate, or transfer. Interrupt your lecture and ask metacognitive retrieval questions to get immediate feedback. Students' answers reveal what they do not understand when they do not understand it. Then, teachers can ask questions on that topic until students demonstrate their understanding. For instance, suppose you ask, "Do you understand?" Students may comply and say, "Yes." Instead, ask metacognitive retrieval questions.

Retrieval questions help students retrieve, understand, and comprehend information. They help students monitor their learning and integrate new information and skills with their previous knowledge. And they help the teacher assess what students are integrating. Students learn to identify their learning problems, so they know where to focus their studies. The novice "student learns to think; the expert student learns to think about his or her thinking" (Quirk, 2006, p. 16).

During a lecture, students do not always realize what they have not learned. Thus, they cannot see where to direct their efforts. Retrieval questions help them experience what they know and do not know. When they have not integrated something, ask more retrieval questions. Give them time to struggle with the material and master it. Struggles enhance their later performance (Slamecka & Graf, 1978).

Table 5.2 Retrieval questions

"What do you understand now if you put what you learned in your own words?"
"What do you understand now that you didn't understand at the beginning of class?"
"What are you finding most difficult to understand?"
"How do you link what you learned today with what you learned last week?"

Giving answers does not develop the student's thinking. Asking questions helps the student think her way to the solution. Now let's review strategies that develop students' clinical thinking skills.

Retrieval Strategies

Decision tree questions: These are the implicit or explicit decision trees that experts use to engage in clinical thinking. Ask questions in the order of the decision trees of assessment so that students learn the steps in clinical thinking. For instance, a decision tree in psychodynamic psychotherapy training might look like this:

1 Where was the patient's response on the triangle of conflict (Malan, 1979): problem, anxiety, or defense?
2 If defense, what defense did the patient use?
3 How could you point out that the patient offered a thought instead of a problem and invite him to share his problem?

In cognitive psychotherapy training, decision tree questions might take this form:

1 Did the patient offer an adaptive or maladaptive cognition?
2 If maladaptive, what kind of maladaptive cognition did the patient offer?
3 The patient catastrophized. How might you help her observe the catastrophizing thought and question it?

In behavioral analytic psychotherapy, decision tree questions might take this form:

1 What was the chain behavior analysis for this portion of the video?
2 What behavior here would be maladaptive in therapy and his marriage?
3 How might you draw the patient's attention to this behavior as it happens now?

> *Principle*: Use decision tree questions to help students move from simple to more complex levels of understanding.

In the following example, the teacher uses cold calls and decision tree questions to teach the concept of conflict.

Teacher: Stina, where is the patient on the triangle of conflict?
Stina: Defense.

Teacher: Jeanne, what is the defense?

Jeanne: Intellectualization.

Teacher: Anders, how could you intervene?

Anders: That's your thought, but what's the feeling?

Teacher: Laura, how could Anders help the patient differentiate the feeling from the defense when asking for feeling?

Laura: That's your thought. If we look under the thought, what's the feeling toward him?

Teacher: Good. Let's go to the patient's next statement in the session.

Questions shift from simple to more complex as understanding builds. The expert sees this all at once. Break down the expert's clinical thinking into steps so that students can learn them. Eventually, the skill becomes automatized. And students learn the steps in clinical thinking.

Decision trees reveal the implicit clinical thinking strategies that experts use. (For more on heuristics, see Gigerenzer, Hertweg, & Pachur, 2015.) Students no longer get an "answer" from the teacher. Instead, they do the clinical thinking that leads to an answer. If they do not learn the thinking strategies, they acquire only techniques. Then, they intervene based on hunches (Peterfreund, 2020) rather than clinical thinking.

Cold calls: Do not ask questions by going through the alphabet or down the row of students. Instead, ask questions from all the students randomly (Lemov, 2021). When you can call upon anyone at any moment, all are accountable. For example, if a student gazes at his cell phone, call on him. Now he experiences, "I have to be present." Then, actively involved listeners in class will become active listeners with their patients.

Cold calls keep the entire class engaged all the time.

Questions to everyone encourage non-involvement by the majority. In contrast, cold calls involve everyone.

Teacher: The patient said he thought the therapist was an idiot. Where was the patient's response on the triangle of conflict? [*Pause. Looking around the class.*] Lydia?

[*The pause creates suspense and excitement in the class. Once Lydia answers, "Defense," quickly ask another cold call question.*] And what do we call that defense? [*Pause. Looking around the class.*] Jack?

Rapid-fire cold call questions make all the students think on their feet quickly.

Cold calls ensure that the conditions in class match those in therapy. If students do a skill slowly, they will fail when patients react quickly. Quick questions prepare students to assess rapidly with patients. Repeat exercises until answers are fast and automatic, a sign of mastery.

Do cold calls, retrieval, and decision tree questions pressure students? Yes. We want that. Why? The student may fear speaking up in class. However, expert therapists speak up, set limits, and think on their feet in therapy. Supporting inhibitions in class sets students up for failure at the clinic. Make sure the difficulties in class prepare students for the demands of doing therapy. Passivity in class teaches students how to be passive, a formula for ineffective treatment.

If necessary, you can grade the intensity of the class by using half-questions.

Examples of half-questions

Teacher: Gary. In this case, the therapist must help the patient differentiate the feeling from his ...

Gary: Defense.
Teacher: And, Jane, you would call this defense ...
Jane: Intellectualization.
Teacher: And Rob. This intellectualization would be part of the system of resistance called ...
Rob: Isolation of affect.

The teacher keeps the tempo moving, keeping the entire group engaged, as they assess the patient step by step.

Here are other examples of half-questions.

Teacher: The therapist must help the patient differentiate his feeling from his ... [*Half-question.*]
Denise: Defense.
Teacher: Given this patient response, Ann, what can the therapist do next? [*Feign ignorance.*]
Ann: Help the patient see how his thought is not a feeling, and then invite the feeling.
Teacher: And the evidence to support your hypothesis would be? [*Teach how to compare a hypothesis with patient data.*]
Ann: The last three times the therapist asked the patient about feelings toward his boss, he kept offering thoughts. This suggests he is not aware that a thought is not a feeling.
Teacher: How could you test that hypothesis? Gary? [*Teach how to test a hypothesis.*]

Gary: That's a thought, not a feeling. If we look under the thought about your boss, what is your feeling toward him for firing you?

When offering half-questions, assume competency—for example, "Who can tell me ..." rather than "Can anyone tell me ..."

Active learning lasts longer than passive learning (Bonwell & Eison, 1991; Bransford, Brown & Cocking, 2000). Struggling with questions means that *the student* connects different ideas, his experience, and his life. You cannot connect bits of knowledge in the student's mind. However, your questions can help students make those connections.

Spaced practice or pacing: The memory of facts and skills fades (Ebbinghaus, 1913/2014; Japp, Muerre, & Dros, 2015). So, spacing or pacing helps students retrieve new information again several times at progressively later intervals (Bjork & Allen, 1970; Karpicke & Bauernschmidt, 2011). Say something once, and students will forget. However, asking questions about that same concept a week later and a month later increases their memory dramatically (Carpenter & Agarwal, 2018; Cepeda et al., 2006; Lemov, 2021).

Spaced practice ensures that students return to content when it begins to fade from memory. Then it has a better chance of getting stored in long-term memory. Forgetting creates a desirable difficulty (Bjork, 1994) because the student must try harder to retrieve that information or skill. The student knows she learned a concept but cannot retrieve it. That extra cognitive effort reinforces the memory, making it stick (Brown, Roedinger, & McDaniel, 2014). As she retrieves that concept, she integrates it with new knowledge, and it becomes richer in memory. Moreover, her difficulty tells her, "I should work on this."

In one study, spacing every three days led students to remember a concept for thirty days (Cepeda et al., 2008). Spacing every twenty days led students to retain information for 200 days! Another study found that a quiz a few days after teaching a concept was most potent for long-term learning (Carpenter & Agarwal, 2018). Teachers may think that forgetting is an obstacle to learning. But forgetting always occurs. Spacing interrupts the forgetting curve to improve long-term retention (Wiseheart et al., 2019).

Teachers often must teach a simple concept again. Why? Students' understanding of a concept changes each time they integrate new information. For instance, their understanding of conflict changes when they learn about transference. Likewise, the concept of maladaptive cognition changes when students learn the concept of schema. Integrating each new level of conceptualization makes a simple concept more complex.

Interleaving: Once students have learned several concepts and skills, ask questions so they can use all of them. Interleaving different skills and concepts helps students understand their differences and similarities. Further, learning increases when students practice various skills together (Birnbaum et al., 2013; Carson & Wiegand, 1979; Carvalho & Goldstone, 2019). Finally, introduce difficulties for the learner (Christina & Bjork, 1991; Farr, 1987; Reder & Klatzky, 1994; Schmidt & Bjork, 1992). For instance, teach students several skills. Then organize a skill-building exercise that mixes the skills. In two studies, interleaving nearly doubled student performance over blocked learning, learning one skill at a time (Pan, 2015; Taylor & Rohrer, 2010).

Or help students use a concept, such as conflict. Then ask questions about transference and enactment to add more conceptual complexity:

1 How would you describe the triangle of conflict? [*Help students think about the concept they use for clinical thinking.*]
2 Let's take the patient's last statement. Where was her response on the triangle of conflict: feeling, anxiety, or defense? [*Help students use the concept of conflict as a tool for thinking.*]
3 Let's look at her conflict in terms of transference. How does she enact this conflict with her father, her husband, and now with you? [*Help students integrate the concepts of conflict and transference.*]
4 When she takes a submissive stance, how does she invite you to take a controlling stance? [*Help students integrate the concepts of conflict, transference, and enactment.*]

Integrating concepts and skills prepares students for the complexity of therapy.

Skill development requires repetition and lots of it. People need to be exposed to an idea three times to learn it (Graham Nuttal, in Boser, 2017). Yet even three times will not always be enough. Think of how often you had to use a word in a foreign language before becoming fluent. Likewise, fluency with concepts requires repeated opportunities to think clinically about different patients. Each time that skill fluency increases, the student's understanding deepens.

Students benefit greatly from repetition and practice, especially when they receive feedback from the teacher or supervisor. Research shows, however, that different kinds of repetition work best for different kinds of knowledge. For example, blocked practice works best for learning perceptual or motor skills (Nathan & Sawyer, 2022). So the rapid practice of a specific intervention may be the best way to master it. In contrast, interleaving works best with conceptual-oriented testing. In addition, interleaving seems to help with discriminating between different items (skills). And it improves strategy selection (when to use a specific skill) (Rohrer & Taylor, 2007). For instance, interleaving different cases enhanced students' ability to identify psychological disorders (Zulkiply et al., 2012).

Scaffolding

These problems embody the strategy of scaffolding. Scaffolding helps a student who is unable to use knowledge or skills without assistance (dependence) to use them independently. Support students when learning in their zone of proximal development (Vygotsky, 1978). This zone consists of the space between what the student can do on her own and what she can do only with the guidance or collaboration of a more capable person. Teachers can provide structure, questions, or prompts to help students learn content and skills they wouldn't have been able to process on their own.

The best scaffolding uses prompts and hints to help students discover the answer independently. The teacher offers prompts as if the student possesses the necessary knowledge. Yet the prompts may be difficult to understand since the student is building on past knowledge to figure out a problem she has not answered before. As the student internalizes these prompts and the resulting knowledge, the teacher reduces the number of her prompts, resulting in *fading* of scaffolding. Finally, students learn how to think clinically, intervene, assess responses to intervention, change their thinking, and become proficient in those activities (Wood, Bruner, & Ross, 1976).

Real problems from actual cases motivate students to solve them. Students can see what they are learning and why. Now, a skill becomes a practical part of doing psychotherapy. They learn when and how to use those skills appropriately in the future. When students participate in constructing their knowledge, it deepens and generalizes, and their motivation increases (Tabak & Reiser, 2022).

Scaffolding questions help students do what they have not done before. Students may not spontaneously link concepts at different levels. Thus, scaffolding prompts help them build a higher knowledge level than they could on their own. A scaffold supports workers while they erect a building. Laborers add scaffolds as the building rises and remove them once it is built.

Table 5.3 How scaffolding transforms learning tasks

Scaffolding simplifies tasks so that they are within reach of the learner.
Scaffolding uses strategies to help students stay on the problem-solving task.
Scaffolding manages frustration by offering prompts to success. Then students don't lose motivation through floundering and failing.
Scaffolding helps students pay attention to aspects of the problem they ignore or don't see.
Scaffolding helps students put their understanding into words. For instance, prompts can help them explain why an approach succeeded or failed.
Scaffolding helps students learn the expert tasks they will do in the office or clinic. Prompts help them use multiple skills simultaneously to accomplish complex goals in psychotherapy.

Table 5.4 Scaffolding strategies for teaching declarative knowledge

Scaffolding Strategy	Definition
Decision Tree Questions	Ask questions in sequence to illustrate a specific decision tree for clinical thinking.
Cold Calls	Call on students in a random order to keep the entire class engaged.
Half-Questions	Ask a question, leaving the last word——the answer——unspoken.
Retrieval	Repeatedly ask students to summarize in their words what they have learned.
Spaced Practice or Pacing	Retrieval at longer intervals of time boosts long-term memory of content.
Interleaving	Retrieval of different concepts or skills helps students link them together.

Likewise, we add, modify, and remove our scaffolding comments according to students' responses. Eventually, they require no hints or prompts.

Retrieval to Facilitate the Transfer of Conceptual Knowledge to Procedural Knowledge

In surface learning, students learn facts and ideas but cannot apply them. In deep learning, students translate theory into practice. What teaching practices facilitate this process?

In the following example, a student relies on an assumption to assess a patient. Decision tree and metacognitive retrieval questions help the student transfer conceptual knowledge into procedural knowledge. In the process, he shifts from a folk concept to a clinical concept of impulsivity. And his non-scientific thinking turns into clinical thinking.

Student: I'm afraid this patient will be impulsive. [*The student makes a layperson's assumption due to a lack of knowledge. He does not know how to think clinically yet.*]

Teacher: Is there any evidence he has been impulsive? [*Invite the student to compare his hypothesis with evidence from the patient. Develop clinical thinking. Decision tree question.*]

Student: It's a feeling I have. [*The student pays attention to his feelings, not evidence from the patient (egocentric thinking). Thus, we help him compare his hypothesis with evidence.*]

Teacher: Okay. Your feeling is a hypothesis. Let's see whether the evidence confirms or disconfirms your hypothesis. [*Invite the student to compare his hypothesis with evidence from the patient.*] Where is his anxiety discharged in the body? [*Invite the student to assess evidence from the patient. Decision tree question.*]

Student: Striated muscles. [*Anxiety in the somatic nervous system.*]

Teacher: And what kinds of defenses is he using? [*Invite the student to assess evidence from the patient. Decision tree question.*]

Student: He intellectualizes a lot and rationalizes why he does things.

Teacher: And is the patient able to describe his feeling? Or does he use disorganized somatic representations? For instance, can he say anger, or does he say he is "about to explode into bits"? [*Invite the student to assess evidence from the patient. Decision tree question.*]

Student: No. He's able to say he feels angry.

Teacher: When he says he feels angry, does he say this calmly? Or does he yell, curse, and walk around the room? [*Invite the student to assess evidence from the patient. Decision tree question.*]

Student: No. He says it calmly.

Teacher: Based on the evidence, how would you assess his impulsivity now? [*Invite the student to assess evidence from the patient. Metacognitive question.*]

Student: I guess it's low. [*The student may have trouble accepting his assessment was mistaken. However, he also may not realize that guessing is not assessing.*]

Teacher: You say you guess. So let's assess. Is there any evidence he is impulsive that we can assess? Because if there is evidence of impulsivity, let's look at it. For instance, does he have a history of acting on his impulses? [*The teacher models openness to all data to understand the patient. Embody the critical thinking standard of humility.*]

Student: No, but he said he wanted to hit his boss.

Teacher: Did he act on that impulse? Or was it a thought in his mind? [*Invite the student to assess evidence from the patient. Decision tree question.*]

Student: It was a thought.

Teacher: Would that be an example of impulsivity or impulse control? [*Invite the student to assess evidence from the patient. Decision tree question.*]

Student: I get it: impulse control.

Teacher: Okay. How would you assess his impulsivity now? [*Invite the student to compare his hypothesis with evidence from the patient. Metacognitive question.*]

Student: It's low.

Teacher: What evidence from the patient made you change your hypothesis? [*Metacognitive question to assess what he has integrated. Can he retrieve the information that allowed him to assess impulsivity? And can he think about how the evidence changed his assessment?*]

Students enter training with unquestioned assumptions and folk concepts from their social backgrounds. As a result, they do not know how to assess patients using psychological concepts. Disagreeing with the student invites a will-battle. Instead, teach him to think clinically through decision tree questions. Then he will learn how to assess impulsivity. Rather than give your assessment, teach him skills so that *he* assesses the patient.

Through decision tree and metacognitive questions, the student learned to assess impulsivity. Metacognitive questions taught him to treat his assumption as a hypothesis. He learned that we need evidence from the patient to support a hypothesis. Previously, he assumed a patient was impulsive. Then he learned the multiple factors we assess in order to think clinically about impulsivity. Thus, he shifted from a folk concept of impulsivity to a clinical concept. Finally, I invited him to think about his learning process (metacognition) to help him integrate new information into his old knowledge.

While decision tree and metacognitive questions help students learn clinical thinking, they make students go outside their comfort zones. Students bear questions to live into the answer (Rilke, 1929/1993). On the cognitive level, if you answer a question, the student does not have to struggle with a question, think it through, and come to her own answers. When she struggles with a question, she makes the connections that will be personally meaningful. On the emotional level, the student must bear emotions that are themselves questions. By bearing those emotions, she comes to emotional insights. For instance, if a patient is abusive, the therapist must bear the emotions/question in that moment. Perhaps, by doing so, she realizes the patient is showing her how she was abused. Now, the therapist can set limits in a firm but compassionate manner, thus, "becoming" the answer by embodying it. Now, she can set a limit with the patient that the patient could never set with her parents.

Thus, we help students tolerate not-knowing cognitively so that they can bear the emotional knowing that will lead to a deeper understanding of the patient. Model how to tolerate not knowing as we gradually understand the patient.

Table 5.5 Decision tree questions to assess impulsivity

A Sequence of Decision Tree Questions: How to Assess Evidence for the Hypothesis of Impulsivity
Where is his anxiety discharged?
What defenses is he using?
Can he say the word anger, or does he say he is "about to explode into bits"?
When he says he feels angry, does he say this calmly? Or does he yell, curse, or walk around the room?
Does he have a history of acting on his impulses?
Did he act on that impulse, or was it a thought in his mind?
How would you assess his impulsivity now?

Student: I think you are wrong.

Teacher: That is always possible. Anything I suggest can only be a hypothesis for us to test. Shall we listen to the patient's responses so she can teach us?

If you are open to students' negative feedback, they learn to be open to their patients. Remind the student that the patient is the true teacher and supervisor. It is not the teacher but the *patient*'s response that tells us whether an intervention was helpful.

Problems based on previous instruction can also arise when we invite students to think clinically. For instance, many competitive students have been rewarded for having the one "right" answer (Tobias, 1990; Steele & Aronson, 1995; Seymour & Hewitt, 1997). Thus, they parrot the teacher's answers rather than develop their own. Decision tree questions teach them how to think based on principles of assessment. Then they no longer react based on assumptions, rules, or imitation.

Other students may ask for simple rules since clinical thinking is difficult. Rather than offer rules for intervention, assess students' learning needs. Analyze their questions. Then we know what to teach.

Student: What should I do when the patient is anxious? [*"Tell me what to do"* = *"Give me a rule I can use all the time. Then I will not have to think about the different contexts in which anxiety arises."*]

Teacher: Good question. I don't know. [*Block the use of a rule.*] Shall we look at the video and see what the patient can teach us? [*By returning to the video, the teacher reminds the student that we look at the data to analyze it. Also, the teacher uses the data on the video to assess the student's learning problem or problem about learning (Ekstein & Wallerstein, 1972).*]

Other students become intervention collectors. One student compiled a list of his favorite interventions by teachers. When lost with patients, he consulted his Rolodex. He knew techniques. However, he did not know how to do the clinical thinking that could guide his interventions. As a result, he could only throw out interventions at random. He did not see the relationships between theory and practice. Declarative knowledge had not transferred to procedural knowledge.

Why Is the Transfer of Knowledge So Hard?

If a student does not put concepts into her own words, they will float around in space unlinked to her previous knowledge. Students cannot remember your teaching unless they integrate it with their prior knowledge.

Students who do not integrate a concept can define it but not use it. For instance, a student can define the term transference. But she cannot recognize it in the patient's words or actions. For her, the term remains an idea, not a tool she can use, a pattern she can perceive, or an experience she has processed. Such students have no concrete understanding because they have no experience using it. It remains an abstract concept without experiential content.

Decision tree questions, skill-building studies, and role-plays allow students to experience a clinical problem. They learn how to use a concept to explore and solve the problem. Then, students experience what they previously could only conceptualize. And that experience provides the content of conceptual knowledge.

Through problem-based learning, students learn procedural knowledge: the skills to use and how to do them. Novice students learn best from simple examples when they lack the conceptual knowledge to solve complex problems. More advanced students learn best from solving practice problems (Kalyuga et al., 2001).

Abstract theory becomes alive when the student has the life experience to which a concept refers. In the following example, a student objected to a supervision suggestion. "Don't we have to build an alliance first?" he asked. For him, the alliance was a "thing" the patient had. He did not realize it is a living, working relationship we constantly co-create and nurture.

Teacher: Let's see. The patient changed topics. Does that help him build an alliance with you? Or does it prevent him from declaring a problem so you could work together to resolve it? [*Inviting the student to use the concept of conflict to understand patient responses.*]

Student: But don't we have to build an alliance before we point that out? [*The student's question reveals he does not know the elements for building an alliance.*]

Teacher: Let's see. If he does not declare a problem to work on in therapy, what reason would there be to work with you? [*Inviting the student to consider what an alliance involves.*]

Student: Okay. But what if he just wants to talk? [*The student does not see the difference between a chat and a therapeutic focus. Thus, he does not know how to think about the patient's statements from the perspectives of conflict and function. Nor can he differentiate his folk concept from a clinical concept of an alliance.*]

Teacher: Let's suppose he wants to talk. As a layperson, you would let him talk. Now put on your therapist hat. When your patient shifts topics, does that help him declare a psychological problem so that we can create a therapeutic alliance? Or does talking this way prevent him from describing a psychological problem? [*Inviting the student to look at the function of the patient's statement. Did the patient declare a problem or offer a defense? Task or anti-task behavior?*]

Student: It prevents him from sharing a problem.

Teacher: And if he doesn't share a problem to work on in therapy, as a therapist, would you have a problem to work on?

Student: I guess not.

Teacher: Well, let's assess rather than guess. He keeps changing topics. Will that help him build a working alliance? Or will that defense prevent him from getting the help he wants? [*Inviting the student to think about the function of defenses and their effect on the alliance. Linking two concepts: causality and alliance.*]

Student: Defenses would prevent an alliance from forming.

Teacher: So how might you thank him for sharing his thoughts and then ask for the problem he would like your help with?

Student: Thanks for sharing your thoughts. Coming back to our focus, what problem would you like me to help you with?

Teacher: Now we see how unconscious defenses can interfere with alliance-building. How is this changing your concept of alliance-building? [*Inviting metacognition: has new information changed old knowledge? And has his folk concept of alliance changed into a clinical concept?*]

Student: I thought the alliance was building if he was talking. But if he keeps changing topics, we don't learn what the problem is. Then we wouldn't have a problem to work on, and there would be no reason for an alliance. I hadn't realized how changing topics would prevent us from building an alliance.

Teacher: Right. If the patient talks about a problem, we can work on one. If he doesn't share a problem, we can't. So it's not whether he talks but whether the *way* he talks builds an alliance.

It would be easy to tell the student how to intervene. But if he believed his folk concept, he would keep letting defenses prevent an alliance. Through these questions, he becomes aware of his role in building the alliance. Now he knows why identifying and blocking defenses can help co-create a therapeutic alliance. His folk concept of alliance becomes a more complex relational, psychological concept. And that will change his work the next time a patient offers a defense to avoid declaring a problem.

Mentoring can generate improved critical thinking (Abrami et al., 2015) when the teacher uses specific questions to explore case examples to address the student's learning problem. The previous student didn't understand how to use the concept of conflict for clinical thinking and assessment. Thus, we could use decision tree and retrieval questions. We have shown how to teach the content of declarative knowledge. Next, we will focus on its structure.

The Steps of Clinical Thinking

Clinical facts do not speak for themselves. Therapists analyze and interpret data by using concepts to discern the patterns that are causing patients' problems and symptoms. To start, the therapist uses psychological concepts to analyze the patient's words and deeds. Next, the therapist looks for a pattern that could cause symptoms or problems. Then she can test that hypothesis by intervening. Did the patient's response to the intervention support the hypothesis? If not, she can change, refine, and test it with another intervention. She assesses the patient's responses moment-to-moment to diagnose the cause of the problems. Then, she can develop a treatment plan to address them. The patient's responses allow the therapist to refine that plan over time. Thus, a more detailed understanding of the patient evolves.

Clinical thinking answers a fundamental question: "What underlying logical process makes sense of apparently illogical psychopathology?" When viewing irrational behavior, the layperson says, "This does not make sense." The psychotherapist asks, "What underlying, unconscious logic makes this make sense?"

Therapists assume that psychological symptoms make sense within a coherent whole. For instance, in psychodynamic therapy, feelings, anxiety, defenses, and conflict allow us to discern the unconscious logic generating the patient's conscious suffering (e.g., Freud, 1901/1989; Matte Blanco, 1975; Rayner, 1995). And we can test our understanding through interventions (Langs, 1989a, 1989b; Peterfreund, 2020; Rubovitz-Seitz, 2002). In behavior therapy, chain behavior analysis allows us to discern the previously unseen logic generating the patient's symptoms (Kohlenberg and Tsai, 1991).

Thus, teaching can never be limited to memorizing facts. Students can find those in books or websites. Instead, students need to:

1 Learn facts and psychological concepts.
2 Use concepts for clinical thinking to generate hypotheses.
3 Form and test hypotheses through interventions.
4 Analyze patient responses to see if hypotheses were validated or not.

Table 5.6 The steps in clinical thinking

Use concepts to analyze a pattern in the patient's feelings, thoughts, and behaviors.
Form a hypothesis to test through an intervention.
Assess whether the patient's response to the intervention supported the hypothesis.
Based on the patient's response, refine the hypothesis, and test it by offering a new intervention.

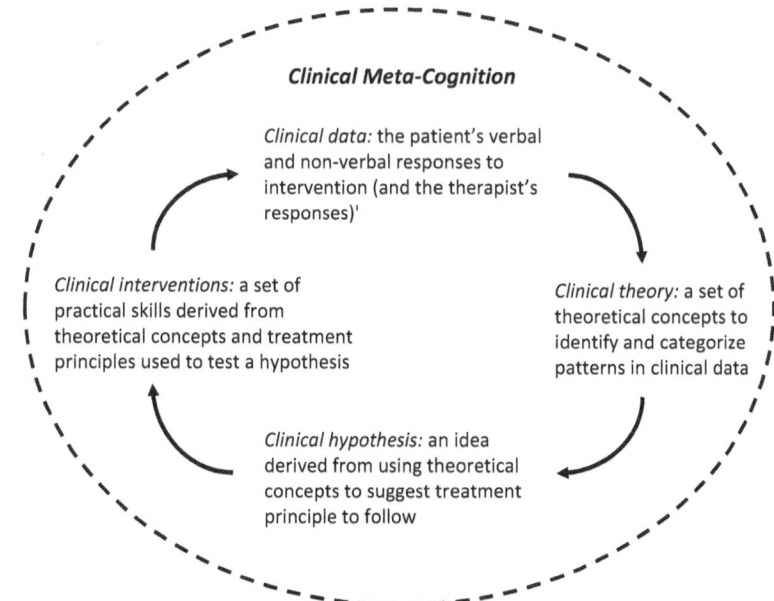

Figure 5.1 A Clinical Meta-Cognition Model, adapted from Peter Liliengren

Instructors teach students to *use concepts to think about facts*. Then they can develop a more complex and comprehensive understanding of the patient. Steps two, three, and four all involve the skills that students learn in order to use concepts for clinical thinking.

Clinical thinking involves a cyclical learning process. First, we experience the patient, reflect on that experience, and conceptualize it. Then we intervene. And the patient's response offers the feedback we reflect upon and analyze. Each stage depends on the others. For instance, experimentation depends on reflection, thinking, and conceptualizing. To reflect, think, and conceptualize, we analyze a concrete experience. Thus, provide students with a concrete example of therapy. Invite them to reflect on it and analyze it using the concepts they are learning. Next, help them formulate an intervention. Then help them reflect on the feedback their patient provides.

The same cycle of learning and feedback applies to supervisors and teachers. Invite students to reflect on and analyze a patient statement using the concepts they are learning. Then analyze students' responses to your decision tree or metacognitive questions to assess the learning need. Then formulate a supervisory intervention to address it. Then reflect on the feedback students provide so that you can revise your assessment of what they see and don't see, what they can and cannot do, as you continue to monitor their process of integration.

How to Teach Clinical Thinking through Concepts

A therapist asked the patient how she experienced her anger toward her abusive boyfriend. The patient responded, "I think he just had a bad day."

Teacher: Let's use the concept of conflict to analyze the patient's response. Was this statement an example of her anger, anxiety, or a defense against declaring how she experienced her anger? [*Inviting the student to analyze a patient response (a fact) using the concepts: feelings, anxiety, and defense.*]

Student: Defense.

Teacher: And what kind of defense is that? [*Inviting the student to analyze a patient response using concepts.*]

Student: I'm not sure. [*Learning need: the student has trouble identifying a defense.*]

Teacher: Did the patient declare a feeling or a thought about someone else? [*Inviting the student to analyze a patient response using concepts.*]

Student: Oh. A thought.

Teacher: And if the patient declares thoughts instead of feelings, what kind of defense is that? [*Inviting the student to analyze a patient response using concepts.*]

Student: Intellectualization?

Teacher: Right. How might you describe the conflict she is struggling with now: feeling, anxiety, and defense? [*Inviting the student to analyze a patient response using the concept of conflict: the relationship between feelings, anxiety, and defenses.*]

Student: She is feeling angry. This makes her anxious. And she wards off the experience of anger by intellectualizing.

Here, the student learns to think about facts by using concepts (e.g., feelings, anxiety, and defenses). Then she learns how those concepts can interact as a pattern known as conflict. For example, in conflict, feelings trigger anxiety, which evokes defenses.

Teach students the steps of conceptual thinking in psychotherapy:

1 Help the student use a concept to analyze a fact (*the patient's response*).
2 Help the student analyze how concepts (*feeling, anxiety, and defense*) allow us to perceive a pattern (*conflict*) in the patient's life.
3 Help the student analyze how conflicts appear in relationships (*transference*). [*These steps illustrate the hierarchical structure of concepts.*]

Facts, concepts, and higher-order concepts create layers of understanding, thought, and perception. Clinical thinking on these levels generates a more nuanced understanding of the patient. And that understanding enables the student to intervene more effectively.

Let's examine how to teach students to use concepts to organize clinical facts.

Step one: The student learns to link the patient's tension to the concept of anxiety.

Teacher: The patient reports feeling nervous and tense. Is that response feeling, anxiety, or a defense? (*concept of conflict*)

Step two: Now, the student learns how the patient's feelings, anxiety, and defenses form a pattern: conflict. Encourage clinical thinking using those concepts.

Teacher: How does the sequence of feelings, anxiety, and defense cause the patient's symptoms? (*concept of causality*)

Step three: When the student can discern a pattern of conflicts, she can perceive a transference. Find out if the student can see a pattern across the patient's relationships.

Teacher: The patient wants to be close to his wife but is afraid she wants to control him. How might that conflict be operating between the two of you? (*concept of transference*)

The student can now analyze clinical facts using concepts such as feelings, anxiety, and defenses. And she discovers how feelings, anxiety, and defenses form the pattern known as conflict. Then, she can assess a series of relationship conflicts using concepts such as transference or schema. (See Jacobs, David, & Meyer, 1997, on teaching stages of conceptualization in supervision.)

In acceptance and commitment therapy (Hayes, Strosahl, & Wilson, 2012), the steps might look like this:

1 Help the student use a concept to analyze a fact (*the patient's response*). "What thought might be creating the patient's rigidity?" "How might you point that out to the patient?"
2 Help the student analyze how concepts allow us to perceive a pattern in the patient's life (*causality*). "How might you point out to the patient the cost of this way of thinking?"
3 When the student can discern a pattern of rigidity across relationships, she can perceive a schema. Find out if the student can see a pattern across the patient's relationships. "How might you point out the impact of this way of thinking on the therapy and your collaboration on a shared goal?" [*These steps illustrate the hierarchical structure of concepts.*]

Retrieval to Foster Higher Levels of Clinical Thinking

Even when students understand a concept, they may not see how it links to other concepts. Nor will they know how to generalize the use of a concept from one patient to another. Scaffolding develops students' higher levels of clinical thinking:

1 Fact-based questions
2 Lower-order concept-based questions
3 Higher-order concept-based questions
4 Questions that link concepts at different levels.

Fact-based question: "What did the patient say?"

Lower-order concept-based question *(differentiating problem and defense against declaring a problem)*: "Did the patient declare an internal problem? Or did he say what he thinks you believe his problem is? Would his response be the problem he wants to work on or a defense against declaring a problem?"

Higher-order concept-based question: "How might you describe the patient's conflict?" [*The student now links lower-order concepts of problem, anxiety, and defense together in the higher-order concept: conflict.*]

Question linking concepts at different levels: "The patient projects onto you, believing you think he has a problem. Is he relating to you, or is he interacting with an image he places upon you? [*Linking the concept of defense (projection) to the concept of transference. Now the student can see how different concepts link together within a theory.*] How might you deactivate that projection to re-establish a therapeutic alliance?" [*Linking clinical thinking to a specific intervention. Showing how theory and concepts lead to practical action.*]

To teach conceptual thinking:

- *Teach students how to differentiate lower-order concepts.* "Is this an internal *problem* or a *defense*?" "Was your intervention sensitive to his *wish* to get well or his *defense?*"
- *Teach students to identify patterns of lower-order concepts that form a higher-order concept.* "As we look at what the patient said here, how might you describe his *conflict (higher-order concept)*: problem, anxiety, and defenses?"
- *Teach students to see connections between higher-order concepts.* "In this patient's *transference*, she views you as a dominating figure. What kind of *enactment* did she invite when she asked you for advice? Now that you see the transference, how do her defenses make sense as reactions to you as a dominating figure?" [*Helping the student think about the transferential dimension of defense.*]

By linking facts with concepts, the student learns to perceive unconscious patterns. Then he understands how feelings, anxiety, and defenses cause symptoms and presenting problems. Next, he can hypothesize how the patient's defenses and transference might operate. Then, he can test those hypotheses to see if they are confirmed. As a result, his understanding increases when we ask questions at different conceptual levels.

Every therapist uses concepts to understand the pattern that is causing the patient's problems. However, compared with experts, novice clinicians spend less time representing patient problems through psychological concepts. And they are less able to add new information to those representations (Lesgold, 1988; Lesgold et al., 1988).

A range of question complexity helps students experience how concepts within a theory are interrelated. Thus, metacognitive questions help the student integrate the different levels of declarative knowledge so she can understand the theory as a whole.

"Is the patient declaring a problem, exhibiting excessive anxiety, or avoiding declaring a problem?" The beginning student might see the patient's anxiety. To promote higher-order thinking, ask, "What has the patient said that would explain why he is anxious?" Now students can retrieve the information they have learned about the patient and synthesize it. For example, perhaps the patient said everyone was out to get her. Can the students synthesize these two facts (anxiety and the patient's perception)? Can they see that the patient may be projecting and fears the projection she has placed on the therapist? When students think about the relationship between two concepts (anxiety and projection), they can synthesize more information into an organic, meaningful whole.

Routinely link theory to practice so that students experience how clinical thinking makes them become better therapists. If the course does not help them achieve their goal, they will disengage.

Levels of Retrieval Questions

1 *Retrieval of a concept (rote memory)*: Interrupt your engaged lecture and ask, "How would you define the term 'defense'?" [*Pause*] "Paul?"
   Retrieval of a concept (comprehension): "How would you describe this concept in your own words?" [*Pause*] "Jane?"
2 *Spacing—a later retrieval to improve memory*: The following week, ask, "When we use the term conflict, how would you define it?"
3 *Link theory to practice*: Invite students to offer examples from their clinical work to illustrate the concepts you taught. "What's an example of a conflict you see in one of your patients?"
4 *Inviting metacognition—help the student think about how a concept changes his thinking*: "How does this concept of projection change your

understanding of why the patient responds to interventions the way she does?" [*Pause*] "Jack?"

5 *Inviting metacognition—help the student think about how a concept changes his way of intervening*: "How does the patient's conflict change how you understand her request for advice?"

6 *Invite metacognition about concepts*: Invite students to make connections between two different concepts.

"The patient's conflict involves sadness over her father's death, anxiety over the sadness, and the defense of denial to avoid facing his death. How might denial be related to the patient's presenting problem?" [*A question invites the student to link the concepts of conflict and causality. When students connect concepts, they learn to integrate information within a theory. And they see how theory constitutes an interrelated system of meaning.*]

7 *Invite metacognition about conditional knowledge*: "Why is recognizing conflict important?" "How does the content of a projection affect how you plan your next intervention?"

8 *Invite metacognition about their thinking*: "How does this new information change your old understanding?" [*If new knowledge does not change old knowledge, integration has not occurred. Ask more metacognitive questions to help the student integrate new information. For instance, see the following.*]

Teacher: How does this new information change your old understanding?

Student: I thought she didn't have much of a relationship with her dad. [*Learning problem: student agreed with the patient's denial because she did not see it.*]

Teacher: So, how does seeing her denial change your understanding of her relationship? [*Metacognitive question.*]

Student: I've got to address her denial.

Teacher: Right. Because if you agree she had no relationship with her father, what will you be supporting? [*Metacognitive question.*]

Student: Oh! Her denial. [*Her surprise indicates she sees this more clearly.*]

Teacher: What impact would denial have on her ability to grieve her loss? [*Metacognitive question.*]

Student: It would prevent it. [*Since she sees the patient's denial and the price of agreeing with it, she will be more able to address it.*]

Retrieval through metacognitive questions improves students' learning and long-term retention of information. Inviting students to think about how concepts are related develops their higher-order thinking. Then they can transfer new knowledge to other patients and contexts.

The metacognitive questions above illustrate how we can integrate declarative and procedural knowledge (questions 3 and 5), new information into old knowledge (question 4), different concepts (question 6), and monitor the process of integrating new information (question 8). Thus, metacognitive questions integrate the levels of conceptual understanding within declarative knowledge. And they integrate declarative and procedural knowledge.

Patients' feedback will fail if students don't understand it. Feedback-driven metacognitive questions allow the teacher to assess what the student is integrating. Thus, always assess whether students are processing feedback correctly and integrating it. If students do not integrate new information, their work will not change.

Also, students will forget feedback more quickly than their misconceptions (Jost's Law) (Jost, 1897). Since new learning fades, repeat feedback continually. Otherwise, students will remember their misconceptions, not your feedback.

For instance, a beginning student may treat his opinion as a fact rather than a hypothesis. To develop his higher-order thinking, invite him to compare his opinion to evidence. Your questions teach him how to test hypotheses.

Student: I think the patient is anxious.

Teacher: Always possible. What is the evidence? [*Decision tree question.*]

Student: He seems anxious.

Teacher: Okay. That's a plausible hypothesis. Let's test it out. Did the patient say he was anxious? [*Decision tree question.*]

Student: No. [*Can the student compare a hypothesis in his mind to evidence from the patient?*]

Teacher: Did the patient report any anxiety symptoms in his body, or can we observe any anxiety symptoms in his body? [*Can the student compare a hypothesis in his mind to evidence from the patient? Decision tree question.*]

Student: No.

Teacher: What evidence in the patient's words would support your hypothesis? [*Can the student compare a hypothesis in his mind to evidence from the patient? Metacognitive question.*]

Student: It's a feeling I have. [*The student equates a feeling in himself with a fact in the patient. Egocentric thinking rather than critical thinking).*]

Teacher: Okay. There's a feeling in you. Let's check if the evidence in the patient's words confirms the hypothesis in your mind. Has he declared this anxiety in himself? [*Can the student compare a hypothesis in his mind to evidence from the patient?*]

Student: No.

Teacher: Although this is a feeling in you, is there any evidence from the patient to confirm your hypothesis? [*Can the student compare a hypothesis in his mind to evidence from the patient?*]

Student: No.

Teacher: What are you learning about the kind of evidence we look for when you think the patient is anxious? [*Metacognitive question to assess what the student has learned and not learned about this principle: assess the evidence for a hypothesis.*]

Student: I need to check if the patient has said he is anxious or has reported any anxiety symptoms in his body.

Teacher: Yes. Although it was a plausible hypothesis, we didn't find any evidence for anxiety being the primary response. Let's return to what the patient said and see what he can teach us.

Decision tree questions taught the student how to assess whether a patient's responses confirmed a hypothesis. The questions helped him shift from an opinion in his mind to evidence from the patient, from egocentric to clinical thinking.

Decision tree questions also help the student see whether his assessment matches the patient data. Telling a student he is mistaken rarely helps. Instead, ask him questions so that *he* discovers where his thinking was mistaken and can revise it. There is no conflict between him and the teacher. However, he may discover a conflict between his assessment and the data. Then he realizes that the teacher is not asking him to listen to her. Instead, she invites him to listen to the patient, the true judge of whether his work is helpful.

Testing students' memory of concepts and definitions does not develop clinical thinking. Take, for instance, the question: "What anxiety symptoms in the body are caused by the somatic nervous system?" This fact

Table 5.7 Decision tree questions to assess anxiety

A Sequence of Decision Tree Questions in the Previous Vignette: **How to Assess Evidence for the Hypothesis of Anxiety**
Did the patient say he was anxious?
Did the patient report any anxiety symptoms in his body, or can we observe any?
What evidence in the patient's words would support your hypothesis?
Let's check if the evidence in the patient's words confirms the hypothesis in your mind. Has he declared this anxiety in himself?
Although this is a feeling in you, is there any evidence from the patient that would confirm your hypothesis?
What are you learning about the kinds of evidence we look for when you have a hypothesis that the patient is anxious? [*Metacognitive question to assess what the student is integrating.*]

question requires only memory, not a thinking or intervention skill. To promote higher-order thinking, ask questions so that students use concepts to analyze those facts. Then, they do the clinical thinking.

Teacher: We have seen the projections the patient places on the therapist. How do they make her perceive the therapist's attempt to explore her issues? [*Inviting the student to think about the relationship between anxiety and the defense of projection.*]

Student: She becomes afraid of the therapist as if he is crossing her boundaries.

Teacher: Then, would projection increase or decrease her anxiety? [*Inviting the student to think about the relationship between anxiety and the defense of projection.*]

Student: Increase it.

Teacher: How might we deactivate this projection onto the therapist to bring her anxiety down?

The student has not merely memorized a concept: anxiety. She has learned how to assess it and its relationship to the defense of projection. As a result, she can address projection to decrease anxiety.

Retrieval questions help us see if students can remember a concept and use it to think clinically to generate an intervention. Students can learn concepts from a book. However, they learn to think clinically when a teacher or supervisor asks decision tree and metacognitive questions. The result you seek is not memory but clinical skill.

Learning retention is best if you provide a mixture of fact-based retrieval and higher-order retrieval. Retrieval questions that invite metacognition improve the students' mental organization of knowledge. For example, when students see the relationship between two concepts (e.g., conflict and transference), they see where information fits on the bookshelves of the mind (Agarwal & Bain, 2019; Sanne Almeborg, personal communication; Roediger, Putnam, & Smith, 2011).

Let's show how to help a student with higher-order thinking.

Student: He said his wife thought he ought to come to therapy.

Teacher: Did he offer an internal problem or an external reason for coming? [*Invite him to think about the clinical facts using the concept of conflict. Decision tree question.*]

Student: An external reason.

Teacher: Would that be his internal problem or a defense against declaring an internal problem within him? [*Invite him to think about the clinical facts using the concept of conflict. Decision tree question.*]

Student: A defense.

Teacher: Exactly. How could you mention that was what his wife thinks and then ask for the problem he wants help with?

Student: That's what your wife thinks, but what problem do you want help with?

Teacher: Good. Let's see his next sentence.

Student: Well, he started talking about his car. I don't know if you need to hear that.

Teacher: Great! When he talks about his car, is he describing an internal problem he wants help with? Or is he describing an external problem? [*Invite him to think about the clinical facts using the concept of conflict. Decision tree question.*]

Student: That's an external problem.

Teacher: Right. Would that be an internal problem or a defense against declaring one? [*Invite him to think about the clinical facts using the concept of conflict. Decision tree question.*]

Student: A defense.

Teacher: As we look at these last two patient responses, is he responding primarily with anxiety or defense? [*Inviting the student to observe the pattern of patient responses. Decision tree question.*]

Student: He's responding with defenses.

Teacher: How does this new knowledge change your former understanding of the patient? [*Inviting metacognition: does new knowledge about the patient change his old understanding? If so, how? Use metacognitive questions to assess what the student is learning.*]

Student: It's a bit of a surprise.

Teacher: How so? [*Invite him to meta-cognize about the experience of learning.*]

Student: I thought he was anxious, but he responded with defenses.

Teacher: How does that change your understanding of him? [*Invite him to meta-cognize about his learning process.*]

Student: I need to deal with his defenses. Otherwise, we won't find out the problem he wants help with. [*New knowledge has changed his prior understanding, leading to a more effective therapeutic focus.*]

Principle: Do not tell the student the answers. Ask decision tree questions so that the student figures out the answers through clinical thinking.

The student can also use monitoring questions for self-assessment.

Sample self-monitoring questions:

1 Am I applying the intervention as I intended?
2 Does my intervention need to be modified?
3 Does my intervention need elaboration?
4 How did the patient respond to my intervention?
5 How does her response change my thinking?
6 What else might I try?

Throughout the session, each patient response offers more supervision, and the student's clinical thinking keeps evolving. Monitoring our work is not a one-time event after the session on an evaluation form. We listen continually to each response from the patient for conscious and unconscious supervision. Likewise, teachers can listen to each response from the student for conscious and unconscious supervision of our teaching and supervision.

The Standards of Clinical Thinking

When instructors teach the intellectual standards of clinical thinking (Paul & Elder, 2009), students learn to think in an organized and flexible manner (Jones, 2015). By contrast, the average layperson's opinion is supposedly as good as anybody else's. Any fantasy will do. It need not match facts or standards of clarity and accuracy. Since many thoughts that students share do not meet the standards of clinical or scientific thinking, the instructor teaches those standards.

Here are examples of teaching the standards of clinical thinking.

Clarity: "Your formulation of the patient's problem is a bit vague. Could you state it again more clearly?"

Precision: "You say the patient is depressed. That can mean so many things and have so many presentations. Could you be more precise about his symptoms of depression? How severe are they? When did they begin? What was the precipitating event? And what defenses are causing his depression?"

Accuracy: "To engage in good clinical thinking, we need accurate information. The patient's husband thinks she is out of control. But our clinical assessment cannot be based on a layperson's assumption or bias. So let's analyze her responses to intervention in the session. Is there any evidence in this session that she has an impulse control problem?"

Relevance: "I understand he is a chess master. How is that relevant to his conflict at work?"

Depth:	"You mention the patient's anxiety, which describes a symptom. If we look at the data on the videotape, which statements did he make that triggered anxiety? What pattern links those statements so that we could find out what triggers his anxiety?"
Breadth:	"Drug abuse could result from imitating his brother. However, if we use the evidence in this session, what are other reasonable hypotheses for understanding his drug use?"
Logical:	"You suggest the patient might be experiencing anxiety due to the election results. That would be a possible sociological explanation. However, what would be a psychological explanation for the patient's anxiety based on evidence from the session? What feelings and statements triggered anxiety in the session?"
Significance:	"You say he had eye surgery when he was a child, which may be an important fact in his childhood. Do we know if the eye surgery thirty years ago is causing his depression today? Given what the patient said today, what is the most significant conflict we could focus on?"
Focus on the purpose and question:	"Our purpose is to help the patient. But the patient does not declare a problem for us to help her with in therapy. So we assess the defenses she uses that prevent her from declaring a problem. Once we do that, she can declare a problem she wants to work on. So as we look at her next responses, let's see what defenses are getting in her way."
Focus on the implications:	"You thought you should confront the patient. But a moment ago, we established that the patient's anxiety was very high. What impact would confrontation have on her anxiety? What impact would that have on how she experiences you?"
Focus on concepts:	"What conflict did we see in the patient's last two sentences? How does this conflict change your previous understanding of him?"
Focusing on the flexibility of one's approach:	"You have proposed a hypothesis based on the analysis of process. What other listening perspectives might we use?"

Summary

We teach through decision tree and laddering questions. Next, we help students integrate what we teach through feedback-driven metacognitive questions. Only the student can make the links between concepts and skills in her mind. Thus, teachers use questions to help her make those links so that new information becomes integrated with prior knowledge. The importance of feedback-driven metacognitive questions cannot be overestimated.

A student *remembers* when she can memorize a definition. She *understands* that concept when she can put that information in her own words. She can *apply* the concept (procedural knowledge) when she solves a clinical problem she has not seen before. She can *analyze* concepts and her knowledge when she breaks down a concept into its components. Then she can describe how she used a concept to generate knowledge about the patient. She *evaluates* (metacognitive knowledge) when she can assess several listening approaches to decide which is most likely to be correct, efficient, or desirable (McGuire & McGuire, 2015). As a result of integrating declarative, procedural, and metacognitive knowledge, she has conditional knowledge. She knows when, why, and with whom to use specific interventions and listening strategies. Finally, at the level of *creativity*, she can design different intervention strategies to achieve the same goal (Anderson & Krathwohl, 2001).

When teaching facts and concepts, use an engaged lecture. Invite students to retrieve their new knowledge and put it in their own words. Next, increase their memory of those concepts through spaced practice. Then, build a more complex understanding through interleaving. Active learning strategies include cold calls, half-questions, and role-plays.

To teach clinical thinking skills:

1 Articulate the skills that students will master.
2 Determine what those skills will look like in the course.
3 Decide what skills students will apply to the content of each class. If the skills to be learned are clear, students will be clear on the task.
4 Use deliberate practice exercises to build clinical skills. (See appendices A and B.)
5 Give feedback on clinical thinking skills.

Scaffolding questions can focus on different conceptual levels:

1 Fact-based questions
2 Lower-order concept questions
3 Higher-order concept questions
4 Questions integrating several conceptual levels

These questions help students learn to use theory as a tool for thinking, which they can test and refine. Now, they no longer believe a theory but use it as a tool for thinking. Next, we will address procedural knowledge, how students put theory into practice.

Questions for the Teacher and Supervisor to Ask about Students

1 What decision tree questions could you ask to teach concepts and skills in your model of psychotherapy?
2 What laddering questions could you ask to teach higher-level concepts in your model of psychotherapy?
3 What scaffolding questions could you ask to help students go beyond their current skill level?
4 What metacognitive questions could you ask to help students integrate new information into their old knowledge?

References

Abrami, P., Bernard, R., Borokhovski, E., Waddington, D., Wade, A., & Persson, T. (2015). Strategies for teaching students to think critically: A meta-analysis. *Review of Educational Research, 85*(2), 275–314.

Agarwal, P., & Bain, P. (2019) *Powerful teaching: Unleash the science of learning.* New York: Jossey-Bass.

Agarwal, P., Bain, P., & Chamberlain, R. (2012). The value of applied research: Retrieval practice improves classroom learning and recommendations from a teacher, a principal, and a scientist. *Educational Psychology Review, 24,* 437–448.

Anderson, L. W. & Krathwohl, D. R. (Eds.) (2001). A *taxonomy* for learning, teaching, and assessing: *A revision of Bloom's taxonomy of educational objectives* (abridged ed.). Boston, Mass.: Allyn and Bacon.

Birnbaum, M., Kornell, N., Bjork, E., & Bjork, R. (2013). Why interleaving enhances inductive learning: The roles of discrimination and retrieval. *Memory and Cognition, 41,* 392–402.

Bjork, R. (1975). Retrieval as a memory modifier. In R. Solso (Ed.), *Information processing and cognition: The Loyola symposium,* (pp. 123–144). Hillsdale, N.J.: Erlbaum.

Bjork, R., & Allen, T. (1970). The spacing effect: Consolidation or differential encoding? *Journal of Verbal Learning and Verbal Behavior, 9,* 567–572. https://doi.org/10.1016/S0022-5371(70)80103-7

Bjork, R. A. (1994). Memory and metamemory considerations in the training of human beings. In J. Metcalfe & A. Shimamura (Eds.), *Metacognition: Knowing about knowing* (pp. 185–205). Cambridge, Mass.: MIT Press.

Bonwell, C., & Eison, J. (1991). *Active learning: Creating excitement in the classroom.* 1991 ASHE-ERIC higher education reports (pp. 20036–21183). Washington, D.C.: ERIC Clearinghouse on Higher Education, The George Washington University.

Boser, U. (2017). *Learn better: Mastering the skills for success in life, business, and school, or How to become an expert in just about anything*. New York: Rodale Books.

Bransford, J., Brown, A., & Cocking, R. (Eds.). (2000). *How people learn: Brain, mind, experience, and school*. Washington, D.C..: National Academies Press.

Brown, P., Roedinger, H., & McDaniel, M. (2014). *Make it stick: The science of successful learning*. Cambridge, Mass.: Belknap Press.

Bruner, J. S. (1961). The act of discovery. *Harvard Educational Review, 31*(1), 21–32.

Carpenter, S., & Agarwal, P. (2018). *How to use spaced retrieval practice to boost learning*. Iowa State University. www.powerfulteaching.org

Carson, L. M., & Wiegand, R. L. (1979). Motor schema formation and retention in young children: A test of Schmidt's schema theory. *Journal of Motor Behavior, 11*(4), 247–251.

Carvalho, P., & Goldstone, R. (2019). When does interleaving practice improve learning? In J. Dunlosky & K. Rawson (Eds.), *The Cambridge handbook of cognition and education* (pp. 411–436). Cambridge, UK: Cambridge University Press.

Christina, R., & Bjork, R. (1991). Optimizing long-term retention and transfer. In D. Druckman & R. Bjork (Eds.). *The mind's eye: Enhancing human performance* (pp. 23–56). Washington, D.C.: National Academy Press.

Casement, P. (1992). *Learning from the patient*. New York: Guilford Press.

Casement, P. (2019). *Learning along the way: Further reflections on psychoanalysis and psychotherapy*. New York: Routledge.

Cepeda, N., Pashler, H., Vul, E., Wixted, J., & Rohrer, D. (2006). Distributed practice in verbal recall tasks: A review and quantitative synthesis. *Psychological Bulletin, 137*(3), 354–380.

Cepeda, N., Vul, E., Pashler, H., Roher, D., & Wixted, J. (2008). Spacing effects in learning: A temporal ridgeline of optimal retention. *Psychological Science, 19*(11), 1097–1102.

Dunlosky, J., Rawson, K., Marsh, E., Nathan, M., & Wilingham, D. (2013). Improving students' learning with effective learning techniques: Promising directions from cognitive and educational psychology. *Psychological Science in the Public Interest, 14*, 4–58.

Ebbinghaus, H. (2014). *Memory: A contribution to experimental psychology*. Trans. H. Ruger & C. Bussenius. Windham, N. H.: Windham Press. (Work originally published 1913)

Ekstein, R., & Wallerstein, R. (1972). *The teaching and learning of psychotherapy* (2nd ed.). New York: International Universities Press.

Farr, M. (1987). *The long-term retention of knowledge and skills*. New York: Springer.

Freeman, S., Eddy, S., McDonough, M., Smith, M., Okoroafor, N., Jordt, H., & Wenderoth, M. (2014). Active learning increases student performance in science, engineering, and mathematics. *Proceedings of the National Academy of Sciences, 111*(23), 8410–8415.

Freud, S. (1989). *The psychopathology of everyday life*. New York: W. W. Norton. (Work originally published 1901)

Gigerenzer, G., Hertweg, R., & Pachur, T. (2015). *Heuristics: The foundations of adaptive behavior*. Oxford: Oxford University Press.

Hayes, S., Strosahl, K., & Wilson, K. (2012). *Acceptance and commitment therapy: The process and practice of mindful change* (2nd ed.). New York: Guilford Press.

Shimamura, J. (Eds.). (1994). *Metacognition: Knowing about knowing*

Jacobs, D., David, P., & Meyer, D. (1997). *The supervisory encounter: A guide for teachers of psychodynamic psychotherapy and psychoanalysis.* New Haven, Conn.: Yale University Press.

Japp, M., Muerre, J., & Dros, J. (2015). Replication and analysis of Ebbinghaus' forgetting curve. *PLoS ONE 10*(7). https://doi.org/10.1371/journal.pone.0120644

Jonassen, D., Beissner, K., & Yacci, M. (1993). *Structural knowledge: Techniques for representing, conveying, and acquiring structural knowledge.* Mahwah, N.J.: Lawrence Erlbaum Associates.

Jones, A. (2015). A disciplined approach to critical thinking. In M. Davies & R. Barnett (Eds.), *The Palgrave handbook of critical thinking in higher education* (pp. 169–182). New York: Palgrave MacMillan.

Jost, A. (1897). Die Assoziationsfestigkeit in ihrer Abhangigkeit von der Verteilung der Wiederholungen. [The strength of associations in their dependence on the distribution of repetitions.] *Zeitschrift für Psychologie und Physiologie der Sinnesorgane, 16*, 436–472. Quoted in Marsh & Eliseev, 2019.

Kalyuga, S., Chandler, P., Tuovinen, J., & Sweller, J. (2001). When problem solving is superior to studying worked examples. *Journal of Educational Psychology, 93*, 579–588.

Karpicke, J., & Bauernschmidt, A. (2011). Spaced retrieval: Absolute spacing enhances learning regardless of relative spacing. *Journal of Experimental Psychology: Learning, Memory, and Cognition, 37*(5), 1250–1257. https://doi.org/10.1037/a0023436. PMID 21574747. S2CID 16580641

Kohlenberg, L., & Tsai, M. (1991). *Functional analytic behavior therapy: Creating intense and curative therapeutic relationships.* New York: Spring.

Landauer, T., & Bjork, R. (1978). Optimum rehearsal patterns and name learning. In M. Gruneberg, P. Morris, & R. Sykes (Eds.), *Practical aspects of memory* (pp. 625–632). London: Academic Press.

Langs, R. (1989a). *The technique of psychoanalytic psychotherapy: Vol. 1. Initial contact: Theoretical framework: Understanding the patient's communications: The therapist's interventions.* New York: Aronson.

Langs, R. (1989b). *The technique of psychoanalytic psychotherapy: Vol. 2. Responses to interventions: Patient-therapist relationship: Phases of psychotherapy.* New York: Aronson.

Lemov, D. (2021). *Teach like a champion 3.0.* New York: Jossey-Bass.

Lesgold, A. (1988). Problem solving. In R. Sternberg and E. Smith (Eds.), *The psychology of human thought* (pp.188–213). New York: Cambridge University Press.

Lesgold, A., Greeno, J., Glaser, R., Pellegrino, J., & Chase, W. (1988). *Cognitive and instructional factors in the acquisition and maintenance of skill.* Pittsburgh, Pa.: University of Pittsburgh Learning Research and Development Center.

Malan, D. (1979). *Individual psychotherapy and the science of psychodynamics* (2nd ed.). London: Butterworth-Heineman.

Marsh, E. J., & Eliseev, E. D. (2019). Correcting student errors and misconceptions. In J. Dunlosky & K. A. Rawson (Eds.), *The Cambridge handbook of cognition and education* (pp. 437–459). Cambridge, UK: Cambridge University Press.

Matte Blanco, I. (1975) *The unconscious as infinite sets*. London: Karnac.

McGuire, S. Y., & McGuire, S. (2015). *Teach students how to learn*. Sterling, Va.: Stylus.

Nathan, M., & Sawyer, R. (2022). Foundations of the learning sciences. In R. Sawyer (Ed.), *The Cambridge handbook of the learning sciences* (3rd ed., pp. 27–52). Cambridge, UK: Cambridge University Press.

National Research Council. (2007). *Rising above the gathering storm: Energizing and employing America for a brighter economic future*. Washington, D.C.: National Academies Press.

Pan, S. (2015). The interleaving effect: Mixing it up boosts learning. *Scientific American*. https://scientificamerican.com/article/the-interleaving-effect-mixing-it-up-boosts-learning/

Pashler, H., Rohrer, D., Cepeda, N., & Carpenter, K. (2007). Enhancing learning and retarding forgetting: Choices and consequences. *Psychonomic Bulletin & Review, 14*(2), 187–193. https://doi.org/10.3758/BF03194050

Paul, R., & Elder, L. (2009). *The thinker's guide to the nature and functions of critical and creative thinking*. Dillon Beach, Calif.: Foundation for Critical Thinking Press.

Peterfreund, E. (2020). *The process of psychoanalytic therapy*. New York: Routledge.

Quirk, M. (2006). *Intuition and metacognition in medical education: Keys to developing expertise*. New York: Springer Publishing Company.

Raney, J. (1983). *Listening and interpreting: The challenge of the work of Robert Langs*. New York: Aronson.

Rayner, E. (1995). *Unconscious logic: An introduction to Matte-Blanco's bi-logic and its uses*. New York: Routledge.

Reder, L. M. & Klatzky, R. (1994). Transfer: Training for performance. In D. Druckman & R. A. Bjork (Eds.), *Learning, remembering, believing: Enhancing team and individual performance* (pp. 25–56). Washington, D.C.: National Academy Press.

Rilke, R. (1993). *Letters to a young poet*. Trans. M. Norton. New York: Norton. (Original work published 1929)

Roediger, H. (2013). Applying cognitive psychology to education: Translational educational science. *Psychological Science in the Public Interest, 14*(1), 1–3.

Roediger, H., Weinstein, Y., & Agarwal, P. (2010). Forgetting: Preliminary considerations. In S. Della Sala (Ed.), *Forgetting (current issues in memory)* (pp. 1–22). Hove, UK: Psychology Press.

Roediger, H. L. III, Putnam, A. L., & Smith, M. A. (2011). Ten benefits of testing and their applications to educational practice. In J. P. Mestre & B. H. Ross (Eds.), *The psychology of learning and motivation: Cognition in education* (pp. 1–36). Cambridge, Mass: Elsevier Academic Press.

Rohrer, D., & Taylor, K. (2007). The shuffling of mathematics problems improves learning. *Instructional Science, 35*(6), 481–498.

Rubovitz-Seitz, P. (2002). *A primer of clinical interpretation: Classic and post-classic approaches*. New York: Jason Aronson.

Schmidt, R. A., & Bjork, R. A. (1992). New conceptualizations of practice: Common principles in three paradigms suggest new concepts for training. *Psychological Science, 3*(4), 207–217.

Schraw, G. (2006). Knowledge: Structures and processes. In P. Alexander, P. Winne, E. Anderman, & L. Como (Eds.), *Handbook of educational psychology* (pp. 245–263). New York: Routledge.

Scott, C. L., Harris, R., & Rothe, A. (2001). Embodied cognition through improvisation improves memory for a dramatic monologue. *Discourse Processes, 31*(3), 293–305. https://doi.org/10.1207/S15326950dp31-3_4. ISSN 0163-853X

Seymour, E., & Hewitt, N. (1997). *Talking about leaving: Why undergraduates leave the sciences.* Boulder, Calif.: Westview Press.

Slamecka, N., & Graf, P. (1978). The generation effect: Delineation of a phenomenon. *Journal of Experimental Psychology: Human Learning and Memory, 4,* 592–604.

Steele, C. M., & Aronson, J. (1995). Stereotype threat and the intellectual test performance of African Americans. *Journal of Personality and Social Psychology, 69*(5), 797–811.

Tabak, I., & Reiser, B. (2022). Scaffolding. In R. Sawyer (Ed.), *The Cambridge handbook of the learning sciences* (3rd ed., pp. 53–71). Cambridge, UK: Cambridge University Press.

Taylor, K., & Rohrer, D. (2010). The effects of interleaved practice. *Applied Cognitive Psychology, 24,* 837–848.

Tobias, S. (1990). *They're not dumb, they're different: Stalking the second tier.* Tucson, Ariz.: Research Corporation.

Vygotsky, L. (1978). *Mind in society: The development of higher psychological processes.* Cambridge, Mass.: Harvard University Press.

Wood, D., Bruner, J., & Ross, G. (1976). The role of tutoring in problem solving. *Journal of Child Psychiatry and Psychology, 17*(2), 89–100.

Wiseheart, M., Kupper-Tetzel, C., Weston, T., Kim, A., Kapler, I., & Foot-Seymour, V. (2019). Enhancing the quality of student learning using distributed practice. In J. Dunlosky & K. Rawson (Eds.), *The Cambridge handbook of cognition and education* (pp. 550–583). Cambridge, UK: Cambridge University Press.

Wright, R., & Boggs, J. (2002). Learning cell biology as a team: A project-based approach to upper-division cell biology. *Cell Biology Education, 1*(4), 145–153.

Zohar, A. (2012). Explicit teaching of metastrategic knowledge: Definitions, students' learning, and teachers' professional development. In A. Zohar & Y. Dori (Eds.), *Metacognition in science education: Trends in current research* (pp. 197–224). New York: Springer.

Zulkiply, N., McLean, J., Burt, J., & Bath, D. (2012). Spacing and induction: Application to examplars presented as auditory and visual text. *Learning and Instruction, 22*(3), 215–221.

Chapter 6

Procedural Knowledge: Putting Theory into Practice

Jon Frederickson

The Purpose of Clinical Thinking: Effective Clinical Action

Good clinical thinking leads to effective therapeutic action. Knowing what to do involves procedural knowledge. For instance, a musician knows how to read music, has mastered an instrument, and can play different pieces of music. Likewise, effective therapists know how to understand the inner music of patients, have mastered thinking and intervention skills, have learned how to use themselves as an instrument, and can work with different patients. As a result, they can analyze and help resolve psychological problems.

Procedural knowledge is not developed through reading a book or hearing a lecture. Therapists need to practice skills to improve their abilities over time. This practice refines our techniques and strategies, leading to increased proficiency and mastery as psychotherapists.

Once students have memorized a concept, help them put the theory into practice. Students learn to translate declarative knowledge into procedural knowledge through experiential forms of instruction. Experiential teaching is highly structured and direct. And it emphasizes testing and feedback (Scheerens & Bosker, 1997).

First, students can analyze video segments and transcripts to build clinical thinking skills. Next, students can do deliberate practice of skill-building studies to develop their intervention skills. Structured learning through practicing clinical skills deepens the student's understanding. Then it becomes "conceptually deep, cohesive, and connected to other key ideas, relevant prior knowledge, multiple representations, and everyday experience" (Pugh & Bergin, 2006, p. 148).

Procedural knowledge is knowing how to do things like riding a bike. It is organized in many ways, but three action sequences are critical: scripts, algorithms, and heuristics. Scripts are extended action sequences. Algorithms

DOI: 10.4324/9781003488637-6

are "rules for performing an activity that rarely change and guarantee the desired result" (Schraw, 2006, p. 249). Finally, heuristics are "rules of thumb that may help us achieve a goal but do not guarantee success" (Schraw, 2006, p. 249).

"Scripts help us organize procedural knowledge and remember steps in a complicated action set" (Schraw, 2006, p. 249). For instance, suppose a patient projects his will to do therapy onto the therapist. The therapist can use the following script:

1 Identify the projection.
2 Deactivate the projection of will onto the therapist.
3 Invite the patient to bear his will to do therapy inside that he projected outside.

This script organizes a piece of procedural knowledge into three steps. Students memorize many such scripts to handle clinical situations automatically and easily.

Algorithms are rules for solving problems that always work. For instance, exploring feelings will be safe if anxiety is in the somatic nervous system.

A heuristic is a "rule of thumb for solving a problem that often works, but not always" (Schraw, 2006, p. 250). It is helpful for ill-defined problems with no clear solution or many solutions. For instance, a patient seems compliant. The therapist starts by deactivating the projection of will onto the therapist. Then, he asks whether it is the patient's wish to do therapy. The patient says, "Yes," but does not sigh. A conscious yes and an unconscious no. That route didn't work. So the therapist asks, "What tells you this is what you want to do for yourself?" The patient makes several non-committal comments and then distances herself from the therapist. Now, the therapist knows that the patient avoids emotional contact by distancing and detaching.

Here, the heuristic is: "If the patient says she wants to do something, but no anxiety rises, this may be compliance. Thus, ask about the patient's will until she sighs. If anxiety rises, her will is genuine. If anxiety does not rise, assess whether the patient is using other defenses."

Table 6.1 Action sequences in procedural knowledge

Action Sequence	Definition
Scripts	Extended action sequences, for instance, a sequence of interventions.
Algorithms	Rules for solving problems that always work.
Heuristics	Rules of thumb that often work but not always

The Objectives of Psychotherapy Training: Learning Procedural Knowledge through Analyzing Transcripts and Videos

Psychotherapy requires specific listening, thinking, and intervention skills. To teach those skills, invite students to analyze a transcript or video and create an intervention. Then, they learn to do clinical thinking that leads to effective interventions. Thus, they learn to do in class what they will do in therapy. Their improved clinical thinking will improve their understanding and interventions.

Further, the instructor can help students differentiate clinical thinking from assumptions. For instance, students may say: "He doesn't want to change," "She has no motivation," "I told her to leave him, but she stayed with him instead. She doesn't listen." These are not examples of clinical thinking. Instead, they illustrate non-scientific thinking based on unquestioned assumptions. Thus, the teacher asks specific questions to help students learn to think clinically.

1 You mention the patient does not want to change. Where would that be on his triangle of conflict: feelings, anxiety, or defense?
2 What feelings or wishes trigger this defense?
3 To what degree can the patient reflect on his defense? Does he view it as helpful or harmful? (*syntonicity*)
4 Why does he view it as helpful? What does it help him avoid?
5 If we assume that conflict exists in humans (*e.g., the patient wants and fears change*), what might he be afraid of? How might he perceive you that would lead him to use that defense?
6 Does his desire to change trigger anxiety? Or is his desire projected onto others, thus not triggering anxiety?

Questions like these encourage clinical thinking and block speculation. Sadly, many students speculate based on biases rather than think using psychological concepts. For example, after hearing the patient's history in a class, students share hunches without links to clinical data from a session. So they guess, unable to assess. Or students may speculate that a patient was traumatized. And then she goes through the meat grinder of a favored bias. But this is projection, not clinical thinking.

> *Principle*: Maintain an educational focus on clinical thinking (the task). And block speculation (anti-task behavior).

When ideas do not have to fit clinical data, they are all "good." Then, teachers reward students for the quantity of "participation," not the quality of clinical thinking. When the teacher blocks speculation, students' anxiety will rise because their musings fail to meet the standards of clinical thinking. So, monitor the class's anxiety when blocking speculation.

Let's look at an example of a student presenting a case.

Student: What problem would you like me to help you with?

Patient: You should ask my parents. They said I had to come or else they would kick me out.

Student: Since your parents aren't here, I can't ask them. So what problem would you like my help with?

Patient: My parole officer says it's drugs.

Student: That's his opinion. What is yours?

Patient: My girlfriend says I have a temper.

             The student stops the video recording of the session.

Student to
the teacher: See. This patient doesn't want to do therapy.

Teacher: That's always possible. Let's examine the patient's responses and see what we can learn. He said his parents thought he had a problem. Was that an internal problem he wanted to explore? Or was it a defense against declaring a problem? [*Inviting the student to use the concept of conflict to analyze the patient's response. Decision tree question.*]

Student: A defense.

Teacher: And when he relocates his awareness of a problem in them, what do we call that defense? [*Inviting the student to identify the specific defense. Decision tree question.*]

Student: Relocates?

Teacher: Yes, when the patient relocates his awareness of a problem onto another person, what do we call that defense? [*Inviting the student to identify the specific defense.*]

Student: Oh. Projection.

Teacher: Right. Projection of awareness. And when he says his probation officer is aware of a problem, is that a problem he wants to explore or a defense against declaring a problem? [*Inviting the student to use the concept of conflict to analyze the patient's response. Decision tree question.*]

Student: Defense. Projection.

Teacher: Right. And when he says his girlfriend is aware of a problem, is that a problem he wants to explore? Or is it a defense against declaring a problem? [*Inviting the student to use the concept of conflict to analyze the patient's response. Decision tree question.*]

Student: Defense. Projection.

Teacher: Where does he relocate his motivation? [*Inviting the student to think about the lack of motivation by using the concept of defense.*]

Student: In them.

Teacher: There is so much awareness of a problem and motivation that he relocates it onto three people. Is that a sign of an unmotivated patient? Or is it a sign of a patient so anxious about his motivation that he relocates it in others? [*Inviting the student to think about the lack of motivation by using the concept of defense.*]

Student: A patient who projects his motivation onto others.

Teacher: How does this change your previous understanding of your patient? [*Metacognitive question to assess what he has learned.*]

Student: He seemed so unmotivated. I didn't see he was projecting his awareness of a problem onto other people. [*Partial answer. Hence, the next question.*]

Teacher: When he relocates his awareness of a problem, where does his motivation go? [*Metacognitive question to assess what he has learned.*]

Student: Onto them.

Teacher: And how does this change your understanding of his motivation? [*Metacognitive question to assess what he has learned.*]

Student: If he projects his awareness of a problem onto them, they'll be motivated, but not him. So, the problem is projection.

Teacher: And if this is a pattern, how might he project his awareness onto you?

Student: [*Laughs.*] Now I get it. Later, he asked what I thought his problem was.

Teacher: And now, how do you understand that question? [*Metacognitive question to assess whether his knowledge transfers to the therapeutic relationship.*]

Student: He was projecting his awareness of a problem onto me.

Teacher: How does this change your understanding of how patients may deal with their motivation? [*Metacognitive question to assess what he has learned.*]

Student: A patient may project his motivation and awareness onto others. And that will make him look unmotivated.

Teacher: Right. Before, you thought the patient was unmotivated. What kind of assessment allowed you to think this through? [*Metacognitive question. Has he learned the steps of clinical thinking that led to his assessment?*]

Student: I didn't think about whether his responses were defenses. And then you helped me see he was projecting. Once I could see he was projecting his motivation, it was clear he was motivated. He just relocated it on everyone else.

Previously, he could not see the patient's resistance because he lacked the concept of conflict. With that concept, he could see the defense of projection and, thus, the patient's motivation to change. Then, he could think clinically about the patient and resolve the misalliance.

The beginning student may feel overconfident because he equates his hypothesis with reality. As a result, he cannot think about or question it, much less compare it with reality: the patient's responses. In contrast, the expert clinician never feels complete confidence in any hypothesis, only in her ability to test and improve it.

Orient the Class to the Task: Clinical Thinking

Let students know what you will teach and why, what they will do, and how you will assess them. Inform students that they will study patient videos or transcripts and skill-building studies. They will learn how to think clinically to intervene. Assess students on skills they develop, not only facts they memorize. Then, they will know what they will do, why, and how.

Orientation to the Educational Task

"This class will teach you how to engage in clinical thinking to be effective therapists. Everything we do in class is designed to help you do that. I will not ask you to do rote memorization. Knowing a fact and being unable to use it in therapy is useless. Instead, you will analyze patient sessions and transcripts and do skill-building exercises. Each day, we will engage in clinical thinking. And you will learn intervention skills.

Every class will help you develop the reasoning skills to become a skilled therapist. Why is that important? The quality of your clinical thinking determines the quality of your interventions. Thirty-eight percent% of therapists are consistently unhelpful. Yet, the average clinician thinks she is in the 80th percentile. We'll have the same illusions if we cannot think about our thinking. Here, you will learn to listen to the patient's responses to see if an intervention helped or not. Then, you can become the effective clinicians you want to be."

Learning by Doing

When students only receive knowledge in class, they never learn to produce it. Solving problems results in better retention than remembering a solution given in a lecture (Jacoby, 1978). That's why role-playing and skill-building show much higher outcomes in learning (Barsuk et al., 2009;

Barsuk et al., 2012; McGaghie et al., 2014; Wayne et al., 2006). To learn, "we're not just copying the information. We're making sense out of facts" (John Dunlosky, in Boser, 2017, p. 26).

Problem-solving does not consist only of cognition based on thoughts. For example, role-plays and skill-building exercises are a form of cognition that enact and bring forth the world of the patient (Varela, Thompson, & Rosch, 1991, p. 205). Through these studies, the student can experience that world, know it, and know that he is knowing it. "All knowing is doing, and all doing is knowing" (Maturana & Varela, 1998, p. 26).

Learning by doing creates meaning. For example, in a role-play or skill-building exercise, students experience the complexity of therapy. They grapple with nuance and get into trouble. As a result, their thinking changes. Practicing skills develops embodied cognition, the experience of the implicit principles guiding our interventions (Shapiro & Stoltz, 2019). Skill-building exercises prepare students for the tasks they will face.

For instance, a student describes a patient who submitted to authorities. The therapist was stuck, but he had no transcript for the class to analyze. To assess his learning problem, I suggested he role-play the therapist, and I would play the patient.

Student:	I want you to tell me what the problem is for us to work on.
Teacher as patient:	Thank you for telling me what you want so I know how to please you. [*When I, as the patient, interpret what the student is doing, the student begins to experience his problem.*]
Student:	Oh. I get it. Okay. Tell me what the problem is.
Teacher as patient:	Thank you for telling me what to do. [*When I, as the patient, interpret what the student is doing, the student begins to experience his problem.*]
Student:	[*Stumped.*] We need to look at a problem.
Teacher as patient:	I definitely want to give you what you need. [*When I, as the patient, interpret what the student is doing, the student begins to experience his problem.*]
Student:	[*Laughs.*] [*Laughter suggests his experience is generating new knowledge.*]
Teacher:	What did you just learn?
Student:	I am asking the patient to give me what I want.
Teacher:	Whose will is driving the therapy so far? [*Feedback-driven metacognitive question.*]
Student:	My will.
Teacher:	And who is in the role of an authority? [*Feedback-driven metacognitive question.*]

Student: [*A look of surprise.*] So what should I do?

Teacher: [*Jokingly*] I would be glad to tell you what to do so my will can be in charge. [*Playful enactment of the parallel process.*]

Student: [*Laughs.*] So I'm one-up, and he's one-down.

Teacher: Fascinating, isn't it! What question could you ask to find out what problem *he* wants to work on?

Student: What problem do you want to work on?

Teacher: How does this learning change how you understand your first statements to the patient? [*Metacognitive question: has new learning changed his old knowledge?*]

Student: I was telling him what to do rather than finding out what he wanted to do.

Teacher: And whose will was in charge then? [*Feedback-driven metacognitive question.*]

Student: My will.

Teacher: And how does that relate to his presenting problem? [*Metacognitive question: can he link the concept of enactment to the patient's presenting problem?*]

Student: His presenting problem?

Teacher: Yes, his presenting problem of submitting to authorities.

Student: [*Pause*] Oh. I was encouraging him to submit to me.

Teacher: How might you reframe your interventions, so you don't encourage him to submit to you? [*Metacognitive question: how does new learning change his clinical thinking and interventions?*]

Student: If I tell him what to do, he will submit. But when I ask questions about what he wants, his will is driving the therapy. But isn't it my responsibility? [*A folk assumption.*]

Teacher: Your responsibility?

Student: Yes. Aren't I responsible for whether he presents a problem? [*An assumption that has driven his interventions.*]

Teacher: That's an interesting question. Can you control whether a patient presents a problem? [*Feedback-driven metacognitive question.*]

Student: I guess not.

Teacher: Unless you are omnipotent, that does seem unlikely. Are you responsible for controlling what he does or *describing* what he does? [*Metacognitive question: can he think about his task as a therapist and the limits of what is possible?*]

Student: Describing what he does! [*The student seems shocked.*] I thought I was responsible if he didn't offer a problem. [*A folk assumption.*]

Teacher: This role of describer surprises you. How does this change your understanding of your role as a therapist? [*Metacognitive question: how does new learning change his old understanding? How*

> *is his folk concept of a therapist changing into a psychological concept?*]

Student: I don't know what to say. I always thought I had to control what the patient did. But if my job is to describe what he does, I'll have to think about this. I don't know why. It's so confusing. [*The confusion suggests the student is changing. A folk concept is dissolving.*]

Through role-play, the student experienced the problems in his interventions. That experiential knowledge made him want to learn more. Further, the role-play elicited an underlying folk assumption driving his work: the belief that he had to control the patient. With these folk concepts out into the open, he shifted to a new vision of therapy.

Feedback from the teacher is one of the most powerful tools in instruction. Its benefits far outweigh many common recommendations made to teachers (Hattie, 2012). Here, a series of metacognitive questions helped me monitor the student's understanding of the therapist's role and integrate that new insight.

A new insight is not merely a fact dropped into an empty bucket. Instead, the student integrates new insights within his old knowledge. The metacognitive questions support him while his concepts and thinking change.

In a class, ask the student and the group to discuss what they learned after each skill-building exercise. What did they experience? What skill will they practice? Metacognitive questions help them think about what they learned and how they integrate new learning with their old knowledge. Further, metacognitive questions teach them to think about what to learn so they become active learners.

Interestingly, when tasks are complex, the quality of metacognitive skills rather than IQ is the primary determinant of learning outcomes (Veenman, Prins, & Elshout, 2002). Why? The more deeply students can think about and understand their work, the more easily they can flexibly improvise based on principles rather than rigidly follow rules (Prins, Veenman, & Elshout, 2006).

To illustrate this dialogical approach, let's compare two approaches to teaching clinical thinking. In the following example, a patient's previous therapy failed, partly due to the therapist's frequent absences. Now the new therapist has canceled a session. In response, the patient repeatedly said she felt insecure. She feels her boss wants her to leave. Her husband has been rejecting her. The bus driver had driven off without giving her time to get on the bus. The therapist told the patient, "I think you may be telling me you are not feeling very secure in your therapy with me."

The supervisor,

Patrick Casement, said: "I think that your patient has been telling you very clearly that she is not feeling secure with you. We have heard of someone who may be wanting the patient to leave, someone who is felt to be rejecting of her and someone who did not want her to be on the bus, so that she was not allowed to continue her journey. This patient has already had to change therapists once. The idea that this second journey could also be in trouble might well make her extremely anxious. She might feel in crisis about her therapy with you. She therefore needs to know that you are really in touch with what it could be meaning to her. It might even mean having to change again to another therapist" (Casement, 2019, p. 31).

Here, the supervisor does the clinical thinking, not the student. But telling is not teaching. This style of supervision encourages submission rather than clinical thinking. In fact, the supervisor falls into a parallel process: he tells the supervisee what is going on in the same way she told the patient.

Now, let's see how retrieval questions can develop students' clinical thinking.

Supervisor: You may be right that the patient does not feel secure. Let's look at this passage from the perspective of latent content. And let's see if we can learn the unconscious reasons she might feel insecure. [*Spelling out the learning task.*] She said her boss wanted her to leave. How might that symbolize her unconscious fear of therapy? [*Can she hear the latent content?*]

Student: Oh. You mean she is afraid I want her to leave?

Supervisor: That's a hypothesis we could test. Let's go on to the next statement. How might the comment about her husband rejecting her symbolize her fear of you? [*Can she hear the latent content?*]

Student: She thinks I am rejecting her.

Supervisor: Right. So, if she fears you want her to leave and you reject her, how might we link those fears to your canceled session? [*Can she connect what she has heard to the stimulus: the canceled session?*]

Student: She might have experienced my cancellation as a wish to reject her.

Supervisor: That sounds plausible. Then she said the bus driver left without giving her time to get on the bus. How might that symbolize her experience of the cancellation? [*Can she hear the latent content?*]

Student: I'm not sure. [*Perhaps stating the question more clearly would help.*]

Supervisor: How might the bus driver metaphor symbolize her concern about transferring from the old therapist to you? [*Can she hear the latent content?*]

Student: My cancellation may have made her feel like I had dropped her before she could feel secure here.

Supervisor: How might you put this together, so she feels you understand the impact of your cancellation?

In the first example, the teacher tells the student what to hear while she listens passively. In the second example, the student learns to listen to the patient by doing it.

Here is another common mistake in supervision. A student has gone over time with a patient. She feared the patient would have become angry otherwise.

Teacher: I think this will create problems because she may feel she can bully you. And your fear of her anger prevents her from facing it in therapy.

The teacher may be right. However, submission to the teacher's prediction does not teach clinical thinking. Instead, we might try the following:

Teacher: Shall we look at the next session and see how the patient responded?

Rather than offer her opinion, the teacher invites the student to form her own by analyzing evidence from the next session. Then she will discover how the patient perceived the ending of the previous session. Rather than ask the student to listen to you, help her listen to the patient. In this example, the teacher's lecture (invitation to listen to him) prevented the student from learning to listen to the patient.

> *Principle*: Do not ask the student to listen to you. Ask questions so that she learns to listen to the actual teacher: the patient.

Decision Trees

Students often start with a big question, "How should I intervene?" Rather than answer, ask decision tree questions (Lemov, 2021) to help students learn the steps of assessment. Then they do the clinical thinking that leads to the answer they seek.

> *Principle*: Rather than answer a question, ask questions so that students figure out the answer.

Break the big question down into little questions that students can answer. Then, you teach them how to assess patients' responses through a sequence of questions.

Student: How should I intervene? [*A request for an answer. Learning need: learning to think clinically so that he can figure out how to intervene.*]

Teacher: Let's see. You asked what feelings the patient had toward his mother-in-law. Then the patient describes thoughts about his wife. Are those thoughts about his wife his feelings toward his mother-in-law, anxiety in the body, or a defense against describing his feelings toward her? [*Inviting the student to use the concept of the triangle of conflict to analyze a patient response.*]

Student: I'm not sure. He does have thoughts about his wife. [*The student cannot analyze the function of the patient's statement. Thus, he cannot assess the difference between a feeling and the defense against it.*]

Teacher: Absolutely. Let's look at the function of that statement. When he describes thoughts about his wife, does it help him express his feelings toward his mother-in-law? Or does talking about his wife shift the topic away from his mother-in-law? [*Help the student see the function of a statement.*]

Student: I see. Yes, it changes the topic away. [*He sees the function. Can he identify it as a defense?*]

Teacher: Would those thoughts about his wife be feelings toward the mother-in-law? Or would they be a defense against describing those feelings toward his mother-in-law? [*Feedback-driven metacognitive question.*]

Student: A defense.

Teacher: How might you invite him to look under those thoughts and see what the feelings are toward his mother-in-law?

Decision tree questions reveal the learning problems to address. Here, the student did not know how to analyze the function of the patient's statement. "Does it help the patient talk more about a difficult topic? Or does it prevent the patient from doing so?" Without understanding the statement's function, the student could not identify defenses.

When students do not see the steps in clinical thinking, they may assume skill in clinical thinking is due to the genius they lack. However, decision tree questions make complex skills transparent. And students learn a map that they can use with any patient.

Sample Decision Tree Questions

When the student needs to regulate anxiety:

1 Where is the patient's response on the triangle of conflict: feeling, anxiety, or defense?
2 If anxiety, is the anxiety regulated (in the somatic nervous system)? Or is it too high (in the parasympathetic nervous system)?
3 Since it is too high, would you explore feelings or regulate anxiety?
4 How might you regulate the patient's anxiety?

When the student has trouble assessing whether the patient has declared a problem to work on in therapy:

1 The patient said there were "issues in his life." Did he declare a problem to work on, describe anxiety, or offer a defense?
2 What would we call that defense?
3 How might you point out that "issues in his life" is vague and then invite him to be more specific about the problem he wants your help with?

When the student has trouble assessing the patient:

1 Where is the patient's response on the triangle of conflict: feeling, anxiety, or defense?
2 And that defense of "my wife has a problem," what kind of defense is it?
3 How might you block the patient's projection onto his wife and ask again for the problem he wants to work on?

When the student is unable to hear the latent content:

1 The patient says she thinks her psychiatrist is trying to control her. How might that symbolize how she perceives you?
2 What interventions are you offering that she could perceive as controlling?
3 How might you reframe your interventions, so that she realizes you do not want to control her but to help her be in better control of her life?

When the student has trouble hearing the process:

1 When the patient asks what you think she should work on, does that help her listen to her desire or your desire?
2 Does her question help elaborate on her desire? Or does it distract her from her desire?
3 Where would her question be on the triangle of conflict: her feelings, anxiety, or defense?
4 Would we tell her our desire, or would we help her see the defenses against revealing her desire?

Let's look at an example within schema therapy.
When the student has trouble hearing the process:

1 When the patient asks what you think she should work on, does that help her listen to her desire or your desire?
2 Is this a maladaptive cognition or a schema she is enacting?
3 How does she enact this schema with you and others?
4 How might you describe the schema she is enacting and its cost to her?

Framing these decision tree questions from least to most complex is a process known as "laddering" (Lemov, 2021). Laddering shows students the steps in clinical thinking and assessment. Through these questions, students learn the thinking strategies that experts use in therapy. Of course, there are many more decision trees. However, these examples illustrate the sequence and structure of questions to ask students. Making these questions explicit helps students achieve mastery. Laddering questions allow you to assess the precise step where the student has trouble in her clinical thinking and the specific learning problem to focus on.

Laddering questions help students see how concepts operate at lower and higher levels of abstraction. For instance, students learn how to organize facts with concepts. Next, they learn how to see a pattern of those concepts. These levels of understanding develop a richer picture of the patient. For example, let's examine a sample of laddering questions for work with a highly resistant patient.

Patient: I was hoping you could tell me what to do.
Teacher: Let's pause the video. Where is the patient's response on the triangle of conflict? [*Can the student use the concept of conflict to assess the patient's response?*]
Student: Defense.
Teacher: Is this a defense against feeling or a resistance to emotional closeness? [*Can the student assess the difference between a defense and a transference resistance?*]

Student: Resistance to emotional closeness.

Teacher: Since he resists closeness, how might you describe the stance he takes with you? [*Can the student use the concept of enactment to analyze the resistance?*]

Student: Stance he takes? [*Now we have found the student's learning problem.*]

Teacher: Yes. When he asks you to tell him what to do, does he take an active or passive stance with you in therapy? [*Invite the student to use the concept of enactment to analyze the resistance.*]

Student: Oh. He takes a passive stance.

Teacher: How does that change your understanding of his question? [*Has new knowledge changed his old knowledge?*]

Student: I thought he was only asking for advice. I hadn't seen he was getting passive and inviting me to run the show.

Teacher: Why might it be important to describe the impact of his passivity on therapy? [*A metacognitive question to teach conditional knowledge—why and when to use this intervention.*]

Student: If he remains passive, we won't get anywhere.

Teacher: And why might it be important to link this to his marital problems? [*A metacognitive question to teach causality.*]

Student: Oh! He takes a passive position with his wife, which is why she wants a divorce.

Teacher: Excellent. So how might you describe his resistance of passivity and its price, then invite the feelings toward you?

This student could sense a resistance. However, he did not see how the patient took a passive stance in therapy. That was the learning need. The feedback-driven metacognitive questions explored how new knowledge changed his old understanding. And they also helped him learn conditional knowledge—when and why addressing passivity is important.

Teaching the Decision Tree

Laddering questions help the student form a hypothesis about the patient. For example, in the following vignette, the student has shown some videotape of a patient, who is struggling with feelings toward his father.

Teacher: Mark, where is the patient's response on the triangle of conflict?

Mark: Anxiety.

Teacher: Jane, where is the anxiety discharged? Is it in the striated muscles, smooth muscles, or cognitive/perceptual disruption?

Jane: Striated muscles.

Teacher: Albert, do we need to regulate anxiety, or can we explore feelings?

Albert: Since anxiety is in the striated muscles, we can explore feelings.

Teacher: Alex, how might you label the anxiety and ask for the feelings underneath the anxiety?

Alex: That's your anxiety. If we look under the anxiety, what are the feelings toward him?

The teacher did not do the assessment. Instead, he used the decision tree questions for assessing the triangle of conflict (Malan, 1979). This heuristic helps students conceptualize conflict. After each patient response, the teacher used the same decision tree. As a result of the repetition, the students soon learn it.

To maintain optimal engagement, the teacher asked different students questions randomly to keep the entire class on their toes. Watch videotapes of your work. If you give answers more than you ask questions, you create a group of passive learners.

Assessing the Basic Learning Need

Videotapes of students' sessions often contain many learning problems. Assess the most basic one and focus on that. Since complex skills build upon basic skills, teach basic skills first. Then, complex skills will develop more efficiently on a firm foundation.

When a student makes a mistake, assess the learning problem (Ekstein & Wallerstein, 1972) causing it. What does she see, and what doesn't she see? Then, use decision tree questions to help her see what she didn't see. Help her analyze what she could not analyze before. Next, use feedback-driven metacognitive questions to help her integrate the new learning.

Students' wrong answers provide supervision: "Ah, the student cannot see the conflict, so that's the concept to teach." "Oh. The student is assuming her warmth will make this distant patient collaborate. How can I help her see that assumption and its limitations?" "She doesn't see the process. How can I teach that listening skill?" Rather than focus on the mistake, diagnose the learning problem causing it. We assess the learning problem by asking decision tree questions. Any question she cannot answer tells us the concept or skill to teach. Then, we can ask decision tree questions to help her develop the missing skills. Elaborative feedback is most useful (Butler, Godbole, & Marsh, 2013).

Let's look at how to assess the reason for an error and address it.

Student: What is the problem you would like my help with?

Patient: My problem? I guess it's kind of difficult to say, maybe a kind of mid-life crisis, but not exactly. [*The patient ruminates and remains vague over the next minute. Either the student does not see the defense and its price, or he does not know how to block it and return to the focus. Decision tree questions help us assess his learning problem.]*

Teacher: Okay. Let's pause. If we look at the patient's response, where is it on the triangle of conflict? Did he describe a problem, anxiety in the body, or a defense against declaring a problem? [*Decision tree question: where is the patient's response on the triangle of conflict?*]

Student: I thought he was getting to it. [*Assessment: he did not see how defenses prevented the patient from describing his problem. He paid attention to his assumption, not to the evidence.*]

Teacher: Did this statement get to it here? [*Does his hypothesis fit the facts?*]

Student: No. But he mentioned a mid-life crisis. [*Student does not see the function of the defense of vagueness: to prevent the patient from describing the problem clearly.*]

Teacher: And when he mentioned the possibility of a mid-life crisis, he said, "not exactly." Did that bring the problem out, or did it erase that as a possible problem? [*Decision tree question: does the statement promote free association or inhibit it (defense)?*]

Student: I see what you are getting at. [*But what does he see? The teacher can assess what the student has learned and not learned so far.*]

Teacher: When he says things like "I guess," "maybe," and "not exactly," do those words get to the problem? Or do they keep the problem from coming out? [*Feedback-driven metacognition.*]

Student: They keep it from coming out. [*Now, the student sees the function of the words.*]

Teacher: Would they be the problem, anxiety in the body, or defenses against declaring a problem? [*Decision tree question based on the concept of conflict.*]

Student: They're defenses against declaring a problem.

Teacher: And what kind of defenses are they?

Student: Intellectualization?

Teacher: He is offering thoughts, isn't he? If we take another look at it, was his answer clear or vague? [*Feedback-driven metacognitive question.*]

Student: Definitely vague.

Teacher: Right. And, if he remains vague, what impact would that have on your ability to get a clear problem to help him with? [*Decision tree question: can the student see causality?*]

Student: We wouldn't have one.

Teacher: So how might you point out the defense of vagueness to him and the price for therapy and then invite him to declare the problem he wants to work on?

Student: What you are saying is a bit vague. And if you are vague, we can't get a clear idea of your problem. If you are more specific, what is the problem you would like us to help you with?

Teacher: [*Metacognitive question.*] What are you learning about the impact of defenses on declaring a problem?

Student: They can prevent a problem from getting declared.

Teacher: [*Metacognitive question.*] How is this new understanding changing your old idea that he was getting to the problem? [*Has the new understanding changed his folk assumption? If so, the problem is less likely to happen in the future.*]

Student: I thought if he kept talking, he would get to it. I didn't realize that if he remained vague we might not get to the problem. [*His folk assumption is changing.*]

Teacher: What can we do when defenses prevent him from declaring a problem? [*Feedback-driven metacognitive question.*]

Student: I've got to address the defense, then ask him again about the problem.

Here is another example of how to assess a learning problem causing a mistake. A student worked with a man who felt victimized and blamed by his wife. He mentioned he was thinking of quitting therapy. In the session, the student asked the patient,

Student: What do you want to work on in yourself that would please your wife?

Patient: I feel like my wife is always blaming me for her problems. [*Latent content: perhaps he feels blamed by the therapist.*]

Teacher: Let's pause. How might he hear the message that he should work on something in himself to please his wife? [*Inviting her to develop a theory of the patient's mind.*]

Student: [*Laughed*] You need to please her!

Teacher: Exactly. How might you reframe your intervention with that in mind? [*Inviting her to use her theory of the patient's mind to guide her interventions.*]

Student: What would you like to work on here that you think would be helpful to you and help you achieve your goals?

I did not focus on her unempathic comment. Instead, I focused on its cause: she had not thought about how the patient might experience it. If we help her develop a theory of the patient's mind, that mistake is less likely to occur again. Then, we can help her understand what she does to make the patient want to quit. A more advanced student would know what to do. In that case, we would focus on countertransference issues preventing her from using her knowledge (Jacobs, David, & Meyer, 1997). However, beginning therapists usually make mistakes because they lack knowledge or skills.

> *Principle*: Rather than judge the student for her mistake, assess the learning problem causing it.

Assessing the Student's Learning Problem

Sometimes, teachers get upset with "stupid" questions. Do not take these questions personally. Use them to assess the learning problem to address. Ask yourself:

1 What does the student see, and what doesn't she see?
2 What is the learning problem preventing her from seeing that?
3 What decision tree questions would help me assess the learning problem?
4 What concept or listening skill would help her analyze this clinical situation?
5 What decision tree questions would help her clinical thinking?

Any student's question may express the group's unconscious learning need. Thus, your decision tree questions help the student and the group.

Decision tree questions allow us to assess learning problems, so we know what to teach. Thus, every student's question is a gift guiding the teacher. For instance, a teacher showed a videotape of therapy involving defense work. A student asked, "Why don't you let the patient say what comes to mind?"

Assessment: The student sees the teacher's intervention but not the clinical thinking behind it. Thus, he thinks the teacher interrupted the patient. The cause? The student cannot see when the patient says what comes to mind (free association) or avoids doing so. Now, the teacher knows what to teach.

Teacher: Good question! We were exploring the patient's feelings toward her rapist. When she shifted topics to her teacher, did that help her say what comes to mind about her rapist? Or did it get in her way? [*Inviting the student to use the concept of conflict to assess a patient's response.*]

Student: It wasn't about the rapist, but why not let her talk? [*The student does not understand the difference between free association and a defense.*]

Teacher: When she explores feelings toward the rapist, we let her talk about that. That's why we ask this question. When the topic shifted to the teacher, did that shift let her talk about her feelings toward the rapist? Or did that shift not let her talk about those feelings?

Student: It got in the way. [*The student begins to analyze the function of a statement: is it feeling, anxiety, or defense? This analysis determines why, when, and how we intervene.*]

Teacher: Later, she said her mother told her to shut up. Did that memory help her talk about her feelings toward the rapist? Or did it get in the way? [*Inviting the student to use the concept of conflict to assess the patient's responses.*]

Student: It got in the way.

Teacher: Here's the fascinating question. Did I not let her talk? Or did these defenses not let her talk about her feelings toward the rapist? [*Can the student see how defenses function?*]

Student: The defenses did, but you kept interrupting. [*The student understands the function of the defenses. But he does not understand the clinical thinking guiding the interventions.*]

Teacher: Did I ever interrupt her when she talked about her feelings toward the rapist? [*Feedback-driven metacognitive question.*]

Student: [*Pause*] No. You didn't.

Teacher: But when the defenses interrupted her, what did I do? [*Feedback-driven metacognitive question.*]

Student: You commented on them.

Teacher: Would it make sense to interrupt any defenses interrupting her so that she could tell us about her feelings toward the rapist? [*Introducing the student to the principle guiding the interventions.*]

Student: I get it.

Teacher: What do you get now that you didn't get before? [*Feedback-driven metacognitive question to assess what the student is learning.*]

Student: You interrupt the defenses if they interrupt her. [*He understands the principle of the intervention.*]

Teacher: How might that be a form of compassion for the patient? [*Feedback-driven metacognitive question.*]

Student: I hadn't thought of that before. Yes, it would be more compassionate to her if we interrupt the interrupters.

Teacher: How does this understanding of compassion change your thinking about defense work? [*Feedback-driven metacognitive question to help the student integrate this change.*]

Table 6.2 The type of content determines how we teach

What We Teach	How We Teach
Learn content: facts and concepts	Engaged lecture.
Use content for clinical thinking and interventions	Experiential teaching through decision tree questions, role-plays, deliberate practice of skill-building exercises, and analyzing transcripts and videotaped sessions.
Integrate content	Feedback-driven metacognitive questions assess and foster students' integration of new information.

Through decision tree questions, I assessed the learning problem and helped him think his way to an answer. As a result, his understanding of defenses, causality, and principles of intervention increased. Then he could describe what he had learned and how his thinking changed. The metacognitive questions helped him integrate new learning so that his folk concept could change. Once that changed, his work would too.

Principle: Always check to see if integration has occurred. If not, students' work will not improve.

Learning Procedural Knowledge through Skill-Building

Good clinical thinking leads to effective therapeutic action by applying specific skills. Yet the deliberate practice of clinical skills remains the exception rather than the rule (Rousmaniere, 2016, 2019; Rousmaniere et al., 2017). As a result, the graduate training of students does not affect patient outcomes (Nyman, Nafziger, & Smith, 2011). In one survey, 76% of therapists said they lack the skills to motivate patients to work hard in therapy. They didn't know how to choose techniques for specific patients (Orlinsky & Ronnstad, 2005). Knowledge of a theory is necessary but insufficient; therapists must be able to translate theory and clinical thinking into effective interventions. Thus, deliberate practice of skills deserves more emphasis in class and supervision.

Students learn deeper knowledge when they practice in class what they will do in their profession (Songer & Kali, 2022; National Research Council, 2012). So, when teaching procedural knowledge, teachers can ask themselves, "What task can I propose so that students can practice this therapeutic listening skill, intervention, or form of clinical analysis?"

Experts possess a wide range of skills (Ackerman, 1996, 2003; Alexander, 2003; Anderson, 2000). However, making skills automatic takes thousands of hours of practice, plus plenty of skilled feedback from an expert. In one review, 70% of RCTs showed that simulation training significantly improved procedural skills performance compared to standard or no training (Lynagh, Burton, & Sanson-Fisher, 2007).

(See appendices A and B for sample skill-building exercises. See Behary et al., 2023, for a skill-building book for schema therapy; Boritz et al., 2022, for a skill-building book for DBT; Boswell & Constantino, 2021, for a skill-building book for CBT; Frederickson, 1999, for a skill-building book on listening approaches; Frederickson, 2023, for a transtheoretical skill-building book; and Husby, 2023, for a skill-building book for relational skills.)

In each class, the psychotherapy teacher teaches some theory. Next, she can help students use a concept to analyze a case transcript. Finally, students can do a skill-building exercise to put theory into practice. And by learning a skill, they feel more mastery. Practicing skills helps students acquire higher levels of conscious monitoring and control. A deeper understanding of the patient results when students practice a skill and evaluate how well they do it (Charness et al., 2005).

When practicing psychotherapy skills, students learn skills, retrieve concepts, and use them to intervene. They translate theory into practice, creating webs of meaning that support and organize what they know. And they experience how the system of interrelated facts, concepts, principles, and clinical thinking works together. This kind of metacognition makes students' knowledge more durable.

Research on the relations between declarative and procedural knowledge has explored four possibilities. Does conceptual knowledge develop first, and then procedural knowledge flow from that? Or do students learn procedural knowledge, and conceptual knowledge flows from that? Or do they develop independently? Rittle-Johnson (2019) proposes an iterative process where declarative knowledge increases procedural knowledge and vice versa (Rittle-Johnson, Siegler, & Alibali, 2001). Declarative knowledge helps students choose the proper intervention to use. At the same time, using interventions deepens the student's knowledge of the underlying concepts, making them more apparent (Canobi, 2009). Thus, skill-building can deepen students' understanding of theory.

Skill-Building as Embodied Cognition

When students practice skills, a bodily understanding of cognitive concepts arises. The student develops a new way of sitting, perceiving, and being with the patient. (See Appendix B for a sample skill-building exercise.)

> *Principle*: To teach deep knowledge, alternate between intellectual learning and embodied practice.

We help students embody a concept through skill-building to learn it deeply. Then invite them to think about what they learned. Metacognition helps students translate their implicit experience into explicit verbal knowledge, integrating their cognitive and embodied understanding during each meeting.

Embodied Role-Play to Build a Theory of Mind of the Patient

Role-plays help therapists shift from folk psychological egocentric thinking to relational thinking. They learn to decenter from their perspective to understand the patient's experience. To build this capacity, invite students to enact the role of the patient, using the patient's words, tone of voice, gestures, and postures. Their embodied experience of the patient allows them to understand the patient more deeply. This can occur through structured skill-building exercises or unstructured role-plays.

For instance, a student mentions patients at her clinic who aren't very motivated. She says they are usually passive. And she feels exhausted by the work. Without further data, the teacher cannot know what the problem is. To assess her problem, he invites her to do a role-play where he plays the patient, and she plays the therapist.

Student as therapist: Tell me what you want help with.

Teacher as patient: Thank you for telling me what to do. [*Enact the problem so that the therapist experiences the problem her question creates.*]

Student: Oh. Because I said, "tell me"?

Teacher: Yes.

Student: Could you give me the problem you would like me to help you with?

Teacher as patient: I will give you anything you want. [*Enact the problem so that the student experiences the problem her question creates.*]

Student: [*Laughs.*] What did I do wrong?

Teacher as patient: Nothing. Now that I know my role is to give you what you want, I know what to do: give, give, give. [*The teacher plays the role to create an experience. Now the student knows how the patient experiences her interventions.*]

Student:	[*Laughs.*] Oh, my God! I didn't realize I was doing that. Okay. Let's see, 'Is there a problem you would like me to help you with?"
Teacher as patient:	I'm so glad you asked me a yes or no question so I could say no. [*Enact the problem, so that the student experiences the problem her intervention creates.*]
Student:	[*Laughs.*] No wonder I get stuck. Okay. What is the problem you would like me to help you with?
Teacher as patient:	I've been depressed ever since my dad died.
Teacher:	What did you learn from this role-play? [*Now, the teacher shifts to a metacognitive question.*]
Student:	I learned if I ask the patient to give me something, it messes up the therapy.
Teacher:	How so? [*Feedback-driven metacognitive question. Her answer is vague. We don't know what she has learned yet.*]
Student:	If I ask him to give me something, the therapy becomes driven by what I want.
Teacher:	What else did you learn? [*Feedback-driven metacognitive question.*]
Student:	If I ask a yes or no question, I give the patient an exit, and then we get stuck.
Teacher:	That's why, rather than ask, "Is there a problem," you ask ..." [*Half-question to encourage her metacognition.*]
Student:	What is the problem you would like my help with?
Teacher:	What are two things you have been doing that help your patients take a passive stance? [*Inviting metacognition about the effect of her interventions.*]
Student:	Asking them to give me something and asking yes or no questions.
Teacher:	And why is that important to see? [*Metacognitive question to help the student learn conditional knowledge: when and why interventions are useful.*]
Student:	Because if my actions are making the patient passive, I'm creating the problem. [*The student can now analyze their relationship from an interpersonal perspective.*]

Through role-play, the student experiences the problem her interventions create. Having experienced her learning need, she becomes more motivated to learn. In this case, my responses helped the student develop a theory of the patient's mind. She learned to think about the patient's responses to her interventions. Supposedly, the problem was her patients' passivity. Instead, her interventions helped create the problem. If I tell her about her unconscious enactment, she may have a cognitive insight. But a role-play allows her to experience the enactment, and the resulting insight changes her. Now, she becomes open for more learning. When students learn an experiential therapy, the teaching and supervision should be experiential. Otherwise, we say one thing and do another.

Viewing the videotape of a student's session allows us to objectively see what the student said and how the patient responded. For instance, a student presented a case she felt was stuck.

Teacher:	Okay. Let's watch the video and see what defenses are keeping the patient stuck.
Student as therapist:	Would you like to look at your feelings toward your husband?
Patient:	I'm not sure I can. What do you think I should do?
Student as therapist:	Well, we could look at your feelings.
Teacher:	Okay, let's pause the video. When the patient says, "I'm not sure I can. What do you think I should do?"——is her response a wish to explore feelings, anxiety, or a defense? [*Inviting the student to use the concept of enactment to analyze the patient's response.*]
Student:	Oh, I see. A defense.
Teacher:	Yes, and when she says, "What do you think I should do?" what kind of stance is she taking: passive or active? [*Inviting the student to use the concept of enactment to analyze the patient's response.*]
Student:	Passive.
Teacher:	When she takes a passive position, what does she invite you to do? [*Inviting the student to analyze the patient's response, using the concept of enactment.*]
Student:	Become active?
Teacher:	What do you think? [*Blocking the student's passivity, the enactment of parallel process.*]
Student:	Yes.
Teacher:	When she takes a passive stance in her therapy, what impact will that have on her progress? [*Inviting the student to analyze the patient's defense, using the concept of causality.*]
Student:	Well, she won't progress.
Teacher:	How would her passivity prevent her progress? [*Inviting the student to analyze the patient's defense, using the concept of causality.*]

Student: She'll wait for me to tell her what to do. And she'll expect me to do the work.

Teacher: How might that be related to her presenting problem? [*Inviting the student to link the conflict in the therapeutic relationship to the presenting problem.*]

Student: Oh, you mean her job?

Teacher: What were you thinking of?

Student: Oh. You mean she might be taking a passive stance at work, and that is why she keeps getting fired?

Teacher: Is there evidence for that?

Student: Now I see how this fits together. Her previous boss covered for her and helped her do some of her work. But her new boss doesn't do that. And then, when she submitted her files late to the new boss, she became angry when the boss called her into the office. She felt he was rigid. But he only wanted the work done on time.

Teacher: Since you are also a "new boss," how does she invite you to be active? [*Inviting the student to analyze the patient's defense using the concept of enactment.*]

Student: When she asks me what to do in therapy or when she asks me how she should handle conflicts at work.

Teacher: How does your new understanding differ from what you understood before? [*Metacognitive question: how does new knowledge change her old knowledge?*]

Student: I didn't realize that when she asked me what she should do, she was doing with me what she did with her boss. [*Previously, she did not see her enactment, now she does.*]

Teacher: Given what you know now, how might you respond to her question, "What should I do?"

The metacognitive questions help the student see where to direct her learning. She becomes an active learner. Afterward, the teacher might role-play a passive patient. Then, the student learns to avoid taking an active position with a passive patient.

When the student judges a patient, invite him to a role-play. For example, have him play the therapist while you play the patient. Then he can experience how and why his strategy doesn't work.

Teacher as patient: I hate myself.

Student as therapist: Notice how you attack yourself.

Teacher as patient: I know. I'm a terrible patient. [*Cries.*]

Teacher: What effect did your intervention have on me as the patient?

Student: You became depressed.
Teacher: How did I hear your intervention?
Student: As criticism?
Teacher: What did you see?
Student: You got depressed. And then you agreed.
Teacher: And was I able to think about your comment, or did that comment become another way I could attack myself?
Student: Right. So what do I need to do differently?

Once the student's strategy does not work, he looks for your help.

Principle: Model openness to the student so that he will be open to his patients.

Next, we could reverse roles, so that the student learns from the teacher's stance of radical acceptance.

Student as patient: I hate myself.
Teacher as therapist: Could that be a thought? [*Defense identification.*]
Student as patient: Yes.
Teacher as therapist: Could that sort of thought make you depressed?
Student as patient: Yes.
Teacher as therapist: If I notice any thoughts hurting you, do I have your permission to interrupt them so they can't hurt you?
Student as patient: Yes.
Teacher as therapist: Since those thoughts are hurting you in our relationship, could we see what feelings might be coming up here toward me?

Then invite metacognition:

- What did you learn about how your patient perceives the world?
- What did you experience when you were in the patient role?
- Did I describe his defenses, or did I judge him for them?
- How did you experience me as a therapist in that role-play?
- How did the role-play change your understanding of how to be with your patient?

When students describe what they know, they develop sharper reasoning skills. Role-plays help the student experience the concepts, interventions, and listening skills you are teaching.

Learning Dialogical Reasoning through Role-Playing

When students fail to understand how the world looks and feels from the patient's perspective, misalliances occur. Role-playing can widen students' perceptions. Through role-play, the student learns to think, feel, and even reason from the patient's point of view. The student learns emotionally because he enacts the patient's emotional logic. And by enacting another point of view, he enters empathically into the patient's world, operating from her assumptions. Thus, role-playing develops dialogical reasoning, the ability to reason from the patient's point of view (Paul, 2012) and engage in vicarious introspection (Kohut, 1971). He feels how the patient feels.

Building Affect Tolerance through Skill-Building

If students cannot tolerate their emotions, they cannot explore their patients' feelings. Thus, when teaching skills, the teacher helps the student develop the affect tolerance to use them. Reading a book or passing a test will not build affect tolerance. Personal therapy is often beneficial. However, the student may still lack the affect tolerance to do effective therapy.

To build affect tolerance in students, repeated practice of skill-building exercises can help. Then invite students to discuss the feelings these skills evoke. Help them observe the feelings and anxiety that skill-building exercises trigger so that they can see how they avoid using interventions that trigger those feelings. Through increased affect tolerance, students can explore patients' issues they previously avoided. Thus, skill-building exercises can provide the deep experiential learning that is essential to doing therapy (Rousmaniere, 2019).

Learning to be a therapist requires us to unlearn social taboos. In good socialization, we help friends and family avoid painful feelings. We do not bring up painful topics. As children, we learn not to comment on others' defenses but to submit to them. However, when students learn interventions, they violate social taboos. They explore painful feelings and bring up painful topics. They comment on patients' defenses rather than submit to them. Letting go of social taboos (culturally accepted defenses) inevitably provokes feelings and anxiety. Thus, the teacher monitors the rise of feelings and anxiety while students learn new therapeutic behaviors that violate social taboos.

During skill-building exercises, divide the group into pairs where one student is in the therapist role, and the other is in the patient role. As you go around the class, listening to their skill-building, assess their progress. For instance, is there a student who floods with anxiety? If you have an uneven number of students, partner with the anxious student. She will get twice as much time and practice to develop her affect tolerance. Then she won't flood with anxiety when using that skill with her patient.

Student: I'm getting confused. [*Student looks a bit teary.*]
Teacher: That can be a sign of anxiety. Are you aware of feeling anxious? [*Identify anxiety.*]
Student: Yes. I can't seem to do this exercise.
Teacher: Sure. It's a new skill. And you're reminding us that learning a new skill can make us anxious. [*Cognizing about anxiety to regulate the student.*] Shall we practice it more so you can develop this skill? [*Return to the task.*]
Student: Yes. Let's do it.

Regulate the student's anxiety and return to the task to build her affect tolerance. Then she will learn the skill and develop the affect tolerance to use it. Let students practice skill-building exercises repeatedly until they are automatized. Once skills are automatic, the student can think clinically while intervening.

Skill-building exercises also help you assess students' progress in skill acquisition. As you go around the class to each pair practicing the exercises, you can see which students have trouble with which skills. Then, all of you know what to work on.

The Objectives of Psychotherapy Training: Learning Procedural Knowledge——Listening Skills

As noted earlier, the folk concept of listening relies on the manifest content. However, the clinical concept of listening involves many different forms of listening. These forms of listening, when taught systematically, help students reach an expert level.

To review, here are essential forms of clinical listening:

1 *Listening to manifest content*: Respond only to what the patient says. And answer requests as if they have no additional psychological meaning. "A cigar is just a cigar."
2 *Reflection of conflict in the manifest content*: Reflect manifest content statically. For instance, "You were angry with your boss. And when it made you anxious, you shifted topics rather than tell him about your wish for a raise." Or reflect manifest content dynamically. For instance, "Although you didn't talk about your wish for a raise, it sounds like you wanted to." Reflect the dynamic movement implicit in the patient's words (Frederickson, 1999; Gendlin, 1998; Prouty, Van Werde, & Pörtner, 2002).

3 *Listening to conflict in the manifest content*: Discern how the patient's words depict conflict (feelings, anxiety, and defenses) (Coughlin, 1996; Frederickson, 1999; Malan, 1979). "You mention your boss unfairly criticized your performance, blaming you for your colleague's error. Naturally, you felt angry (*feeling*). And the anger made you uncomfortable (*anxiety*). Then you began to second-guess yourself (*defense*) and got depressed (*resulting symptom*). I wonder if second-guessing yourself was a way to turn anger onto yourself and protect your boss instead."

4 *Listening to conflict in the process*: Discerning how the sequence of the patient's associations illustrates conflict. For instance, how long can the patient talk freely about a topic before a sentence inhibits that flow? (A. Freud, 1936; Davison, Bristol, & Pray, 1986; Davison, Pray, & Bristol, 1990; Gray, 1994).

5 *Listening to conflict in the latent content*: Discerning how the symbolic meanings of the patient's words depict conflict. How might the patient's words symbolize her unconscious experience of the therapist? If the patient frequently complains that others try to dominate her, is it possible she perceives you similarly? (Frederickson, 1999; Gill, 1983a, 1983b; Langs, 1989a, 1989b; Raney, 1983; Smith, 2018).

6 *Listening to conflict in the enactment*: Discerning how the therapist and the patient unconsciously enact the conflict (Fiscalini, 2004; Langs, 1989a, 1989b; Levenson, 1972, 1984, 1991). For instance, a patient who fears asserting herself in relationships hides her wishes by agreeing with the opinions of others. In therapy, the therapist might make a suggestion, and the patient complies with him and agrees.

7 *Listening to conflict in the countertransference*: Discerning how the therapist's feelings and thoughts may symbolize an aspect of the patient's conflict in the transference or conflicts in the therapist (Ogden, 1992; Racker, 1968).

To develop listening skills, invite students to use one of these listening approaches to analyze a session transcript. Then, they learn to see the unconscious logic of the patient's words and behaviors.

Inviting the Class to Analyze a Transcript

In the following example, the teacher asks questions to teach the class how to listen to latent content in a transcript they are analyzing.

T (Therapist): So you have an appointment Monday? Your next psychiatry appointment?

P (Patient): Yeah, and I don't want to go. I don't know what the point of going is. What are we gonna talk about? I'm going to sit there. For an hour. Rocking. There's nothing to talk about with him. I really don't like my psychiatrist.

Teacher: The patient says, "I don't know what the point of going is. There's nothing to talk about with him. I really don't like my psychiatrist." How might that symbolize the patient's perception of the therapist? [*Helping the student listen for latent content.*]

Jane: That she doesn't want to talk with the therapist?

Teacher: Right. And how might she feel about the therapist if we listen to the latent content?

Jim: She doesn't like the therapist.

Teacher: Right. Let's keep listening and see if the latent content supports that hypothesis. [*The teacher continues by reading the following transcript.*]

T: Yeah. So you go on Monday and fill out the provider change request card and get the injection. If you want to talk about lowering the dose or switching to pills rather than your injection, you can do that. Any number of things you can bring up at the appointment. You mentioned several things to me you might like to discuss.

P: And what if he says no? Like, don't I have a say in what happens to my own body?

Teacher: "Don't I have a say in what happens to my body?" If we listen to the latent content, how might the patient perceive her therapist?

Terry: Like maybe she thinks the therapist wants to say what happens with her body.

Teacher: Let's see how the therapist handles that.

T: Sure, of course. If he says no to anything, you can ask him to explain why it is a no. You can ask questions, and his job is to help you understand why the answer is no. So instead of just hearing no, you can get an explanation and have a conversation about it.

P: [*Long pause*] I really don't like him. [*Begins rocking back and forth.*]

Teacher: If we listen to the latent content, how might she perceive the therapist?

Tom: She doesn't like him.

Teacher: That's very possible. Let's keep listening to the latent content and see what else we can learn.

T: Yeah, yes. And you have something you want [a specific medication for ADHD], and it is not happening.

P: It hasn't been happening. I've been asking him since June for the same thing, and he hasn't done shit about it. And the only reason I'm off all my other meds is because I did that myself. He was not thrilled with me when I did that.

Teacher: If we listen to the latent content, how might the patient perceive the therapist here?

Jane: It sounds like she has been wanting something from the therapist, and he hasn't given it.

Teacher: Yes. And if you look at the latent content of her last sentence, how might she perceive the therapist?

Lena: She thinks he is not thrilled with her decision to go off her medications.

Teacher: And if she has gone off her other medications, what else might she be thinking of stopping?

Jane: Therapy.

Teacher: Exactly. Often when patients say they have side effects to medications, they are having side effects to the therapist. Let's listen some more to the latent content to see what else we can learn.

T: Yup, the two of you disagree on things.

P: A lot of things. I'm a very stubborn person. When I have something in my head, it's there and not going away.

T: Yup, I've noticed that.

P: [*Laughter*] When I'm on a mission, I'm on a mission.

T: Yup, mmhmm. And that can be a positive, a strength of yours. When you have got something in your focus, you are able to stick to it.

P: Yeah, I wish it worked that way with school.

Teacher: If we listen to the latent content of her last sentence, how might she perceive the therapy?

Alex: Something is not working in therapy.

Teacher: Any sense what that is, based on what she said here?

Marie: She said they disagree on a lot of things.

Teacher: So what might not be working in therapy?

Marie: Maybe she thinks it doesn't work in therapy when she disagrees with the therapist.

Teacher: Let's listen some more to the latent content to see if there is evidence for that.

T: So, did you notice that as we were talking about psychiatry and it seemed like you were getting angry, or frustrated, you started to rock back and forth? Did you notice that connection?

P: [*Shakes her head.*] Mm-mmm.

T: Yeah, so I guess I did, and I wondered if you did as well. That as some anger came up as we talked about psychiatry you weren't rocking at all and then started to rock as some anger came up. Did you notice that?

P: I was trying to calm myself down.

T: Right, yeah exactly, and trying to calm yourself down because what feelings were you having?

P: A lot of anger. Wanting to go off, again, on him but realizing there is no point of it.

Teacher: As we listen to the latent content in these last two sentences, how might she feel toward the therapist?

Jack: She's angry.

Teacher: And what else could she be telling us when we listen to the latent content?

Jane: She doesn't see any point in telling him about her anger.

Teacher: Right. So if she perceives him that way, will she reach out to him for help with her anxiety, or will she try to handle it herself?

Jane: She'll handle it herself because she is afraid of him.

Teacher: That sounds very plausible. Let's listen some more to the latent content to see what she can teach us.

T: Yeah, and you are here with me so you could go off on the psychiatrist, but it's just me who is here. But there was something about anger coming up now, and you wanted to calm that down, so you started moving, rocking back and forth, which is what you've described to me before when you can't sit still. And it seems like maybe it is happening in this moment, too. Happening right now? Moving a little bit?

P: I've been rocking my feet this whole time.

T: And the rocking I could see started happening as we were talking about psychiatry.

P: Oh, well. I just, I don't like him. That's all I can say. He has rubbed me the wrong way since the beginning. I thought I was stuck with him.

Teacher: As we listen to the latent content in the last sentence, how else could she perceive the therapist? Tom?

Tom: She feels stuck with him.

Teacher: This is important, isn't it! When patients feel stuck and angry, able to talk about this only symbolically, that can be a sign they are ready to drop out. So we want to understand why she is angry with the therapist, so she doesn't drop out of treatment. Let's see what unconscious supervision the patient can give us.

T: Right, yeah. And so you've told me in the past about being unable to sit still, rocking back and forth, is an issue for you, it bothers you, it makes it hard to get work done. We've talked a little bit about what happens in those moments, but not much. But I think what caught my attention today in being with you was that as I sensed some anger coming up, I could also see you were rocking. Which I thought was interesting and something for us to notice together to maybe help you understand yourself a little bit better. These moments where you can't sit still it seems like, at least today here with me, it was a behavior you started to do to manage anger coming up. Kind of gives a reason for the rocking in a new sense, like there is a reason you would rock, right? Like to deal with a feeling?

P: [*nodding, pause*] Probably, yeah. Like from when I was a kid. Cause my mom was abusive, very abusive to me. And um ... I was never allowed to fight back. I just had to take it.

Teacher: If we listen to the latent content in her comments about her mom, how might she be unconsciously perceiving the therapist's recent interventions?

Marie: She perceives the therapist as abusive. That she can't fight back and must take it.

Teacher: If she perceives the therapist that way, that would certainly explain her anger, wouldn't it? Let's listen some more to the latent content.

T: Yeah, so you couldn't fight back. You had to take it.

P: I wasn't allowed to stand up for myself verbally, or I got the shit beat out of me.

Teacher: If we listen to the latent content, how might she perceive the therapist? Jennie?

Jennie: I'm not allowed to stand up for myself verbally in therapy. Or else you will beat me up?

Teacher: Apparently, something has happened in therapy to make the patient believe she is not allowed to stand up for herself in therapy and she might be punished for doing so.

In this model of teaching, the students actively listen and interpret, learning by doing. In this example, the task is learning to listen to latent content. So the teacher's question remains the same throughout. "If we listen to the latent content, on an unconscious level, how might the patient experience the therapist's intervention?" If one student has difficulties, we might focus more on him. However, if he is learning well, we might rely more on cold calls to the entire class to keep everyone involved. Or if the student is a bit anxious, the teacher can ask the group more questions to reduce the focus on the student and, thus, lessen his anxiety. (See Appendix A, which shows how to use this material for a test to assess students' listening and analytic skills.)

Commentary

Skill-building studies allow the teacher to measure the student's mastery. Thus, to teach a listening skill, you can use decision tree questions with a transcript. You can do skill-building exercises for that skill. And you can design tests to assess students' mastery. Approaching skill-building from several perspectives helps solidify students' mastery of the skills. And their clinical thinking will become more complex and nuanced.

Problem-based learning builds students' critical thinking capacities (Haobin et al., 2008). When students learn to listen from several perspectives, they integrate different strands of evidence within a holistic understanding. And they can think about the strengths and limitations of each mode of listening (Tansey & Burke, 1995). The capacity for metacognition is another marker for expert clinical listening.

Each listening perspective shapes how we hear and the meanings we find. No listening perspective is neutral. If we can listen from only one approach, our perception becomes hostage to that tool. Instead, we can use several listening approaches to gain perspective on how we listen to and understand the patient. Then we can avoid the danger of making a hypothesis based on only one perspective. By listening from many perspectives, students can compare them. Then they can detect the unconscious conflicts driving the patient's problems so that they can formulate targeted interventions.

It is not enough for students to know when an intervention did not help. If they understand *why (conditional knowledge)*, they won't make the same mistake again. Diagnose why they made a mistake so that you can teach them better strategies to use in the future. Learning occurs more rapidly when feedback is provided (Lhyle & Kulhavy, 1987). And immediate feedback promotes learning more than delayed feedback (Pressley & McCormick, 1995). Explain why correct responses are reasonable and incorrect answers are not (Bangert-Drowns et al., 1991). Feedback on a pattern of errors is more valuable than feedback on an individual mistake. Instructional feedback explains what to improve and how to improve. For instance, address students' misconceptions, misunderstandings, and problems with their clinical thinking (Hattie, 2012; Vardi, 2015). Feedback, when an idea is wrong, can help students reformulate a concept at a new and higher level.

After providing feedback, teachers can use metacognitive questions to assess how students integrated the feedback. For example, you might give the class a session transcript and ask them to figure out the triangle of conflict. Or you might ask them to describe the transference based on the latent content. You might ask them to identify the defenses in the transcript. Then ask them to describe how the defenses create the patient's presenting problems. Or you might ask the students which therapist interventions blocked the therapy.

You might ask students to assess the therapist's therapeutic focus.

* When did the therapist lose her therapeutic focus?
* How would you intervene at that moment to re-establish a clear therapeutic focus?
* Does the therapist reference what the patient says or what the therapist thinks?
* Where is the therapist focusing, and does the evidence support that focus?
* How do the patient's responses help us understand her difficulties more clearly?

Conclusion

To develop procedural knowledge, students study videotaped sessions or session transcripts. They learn how to use concepts and listening skills to analyze sessions. And they engage in the deliberate practice of skill-building exercises. Students learn procedural knowledge best through experiential exercises. We learn through experience (Bion, 1962). Hence, we use an experiential model of supervision and teaching.

The expert possesses extensive procedural knowledge, organized through scripts, algorithms, and heuristics. With those skills, she can develop a conceptual model of the problem to solve it. However, deliberate practice of procedural knowledge is necessary to make specific skills automatic. Then, the student can reflect on their implicit patterns and principles. As a result, the student understands how, when, and why we intervene.

Questions for the Teacher and Supervisor to Ask about the Student

Procedural knowledge questions are designed to elicit steps/processes in implementing concepts, skills, and interventions, answering the question, "How do you turn your clinical thinking into effective interventions?"

* What decision tree questions could you ask to help students turn their clinical thinking into interventions?
* What laddering questions could you ask to help students formulate interventions at different conceptual levels (e.g., defense, transference, enactment, and countertransference)?
* What metacognitive questions could you ask to help students integrate experiential knowledge from skill-building exercises?

References

Ackerman, P. (1996). A theory of adult intellectual development: Process, personality, interests, and knowledge. *Intelligence, 22*, 227–257. https://doi.org/10.1016/S0160-2896(96)90016-1

Ackerman, P. (2003). Cognitive ability and non-ability traits of expertise. *Educational Researcher, 32*, 15–20.

Alexander, P. (2003). The development of expertise: The journey from acclimation to proficiency. *Educational Researcher, 32*, 10–14.

Anderson, J. (2000). *Learning and memory: An integrated approach* (2nd ed.). Hoboken, N. J.: John Wiley & Sons Inc.

Bangert-Drowns, R., Kulik, C., Kulik, J., & Morgan, M. (1991). The instructional effect of feedback in test-like events. *Review of Educational Research, 61*, 213–238.

Barsuk, J., Cohen, E., Vosenilek, J., O'Connor, L., McGaghie, W., & Wayne, D. (2012). Simulation-based education with mastery learning improves parencentesis skills. *Journal of Graduate Medical Education, 4*, 21–27.

Barsuk, J., McGaghie, W., Cohen, E., Balachandran, J., & Wayne, D. (2009). Use of simulation-based mastery learning to improve the quality of central venous catheter placement in a medical intensive care unit. *Journal of Hospital Medicine, 4*, 397–403.

Behary, W., Farrell, J., Vaz, A., & Rousmaniere, T. (2023). *Deliberate practice in schema therapy*. Washington, D.C.: APA Press.

Bion, W. R. (1962). *Learning from experience*. London: William Heinemann.

Boritz, T., McCain, S., Vaz, A., & Rousmaniere, T. (2022). *Deliberate practice in DBT*. Washington, D.C.: APA Press.

Boser, U. (2017). *Learn better: Mastering the skills for success in life, business, and school, or How to become an expert in just about anything*. New York: Rodale Books.

Boswell, J., & Constantino, M. (2021). *Deliberate practice in cognitive behavioral therapy*. Washington, D.C.: APA Press.

Butler, A., Godbole, N., & Marsh, E. (2013). Explanation feedback is better than correct answer feedback for promoting transfer of learning. *Journal of Educational Psychology, 105*(2), 290–298.

Canobi, K. (2009). Concept-procedure interactions in children's addition and subtraction. *Journal of Experimental Child Psychology, 102*, 131–149.

Casement, P. (2019). *Learning along the way: Further reflections on psychoanalysis and psychotherapy*. New York: Routledge.

Charness, N., Tuffiash, M., Kramp, R., & Reingold, E. (2005). The role of deliberate practice in chess. *Applied Cognitive Psychology, 19*(2), 151–165. https://doi.org/10.1002/Acp.1106

Coughlin, P. (1996). *Intensive short term dynamic psychotherapy*. New York: Wiley.

Davison, W. T., Bristol, C., & Pray, M. (1986). Turning aggression on the self: A study of psychoanalytic process. *The Psychoanalytic Quarterly, 55*(2), 273–295.

Davison, W. T., Pray, M., & Bristol, C. (1990). Mutative interpretation and close process monitoring in a study of psychoanalytic process. *The Psychoanalytic Quarterly, 59*(4), 599–628.

Ekstein, R., & Wallerstein, R. (1972). *The teaching and learning of psychotherapy* (2nd ed.). New York: International Universities Press.

Fiscalini, J. (2004). *Coparticipant psychoanalysis: Toward a new theory of clinical inquiry.* New York: Columbia University Press.

Frederickson, J. (1999). *Psychodynamic psychotherapy: Listening from multiple perspectives.* New York: Routledge.

Frederickson, J. (2023). *Healing through relating: A skill-building book for therapists.* Kensington, Md.: Seven Leaves Press.

Freud, A. (1936). *The ego and the mechanisms of defense.* New York: Norton.

Gendlin, E. (1998). *Focusing-oriented psychotherapy: A manual of the experiential method.* New York: Guilford Press.

Gill, M., & Hoffman, I. (1983a). *Analysis of transference, Vol. 1.* New York: International Universities Press.

Gill, M., & Hoffman, I. (1983b). *Analysis of transference, Vol. 2.* New York: International Universities Press.

Gray, P. (1994). *The ego and the analysis of defense.* New York: Aronson.

Haobin, Y., Wipada, K., Areewan, K., & Williams, B. (2008). Promoting thinking skills through problem-based learning. *Journal of Social Science and Humanities, 2*(2), 85–100.

Hattie, J. (2012). *Visible learning: A synthesis of over 800 meta-analyses relating to achievement.* London: Routledge.

Husby, V. (2023). *Targeted skills training: Relational skills in psychotherapy.* Oslo: Gyldenhal.

Jacobs, D., David, P., & Meyer, D. (1997). *The supervisory encounter: A guide for teachers of psychodynamic psychotherapy and psychoanalysis.* New Haven, Conn.: Yale University Press.

Jacoby, L. (1978). On interpreting the effects of repetition: Solving a problem versus remembering a solution. *Journal of Verbal Learning and Verbal Behavior, 17,* 649–667.

Kohut, H. (1971). *The analysis of the self: A systematic approach to the psychoanalytic treatment of narcissistic personality disorders.* New York: International Universities Press.

Langs, R. (1989a). *The technique of psychoanalytic psychotherapy: Vol. 1. Initial contact: Theoretical framework: Understanding the patient's communications: The therapist's interventions.* New York: Aronson.

Langs, R. (1989b). *The technique of psychoanalytic psychotherapy: Vol. 2. Responses to interventions: Patient-therapist relationship: Phases of psychotherapy.* New York: Aronson.

Lemov, D. (2021). *Teach like a champion 3.0.* New York: Jossey-Bass.

Levenson, E. (1972). *The fallacy of understanding.* New York: Basic Books.

Levenson, E. (1984). *The ambiguity of change: An inquiry into the nature of psychoanalytic reality.* New York: Basic Books.

Levenson, E. (1991). *The purloined self: Interpersonal perspectives in psychoanalysis.* New York: Contemporary Psychoanalytic Books.

Lhyle, K., & Kulhavy, R. (1987). Feedback processing and error correction. *Journal of Educational Psychology, 79,* 320–322.

Lynagh, M., Burton, R., & Sanson-Fisher, R. (2007). A systematic review of medical skills laboratory training: Where to from here? *Medical Education*, *41*(9), 879–887.

Malan, D. (1979). *Individual psychotherapy and the science of psychodynamics* (2nd ed.). London: Butterworth-Heineman.

Manning, B. & Payne, B. (1996). *Self-talk for teachers and students*. Allyn & Bacon: Needham.

Maturana, H., & Varela, F. (1998). *The tree of knowledge: The biological roots of human understanding*. Boston, Mass.: Shambhala Publications.

McGaghie, W., Issenberg, S., Barsuk, J., & Wayne, D. (2014). A critical review of simulation-based mastery learning with translational outcomes. *Medical Education*, *48*, 375–385.

National Research Council. (2012). *A framework for K-12 science education: Practices, crosscutting concepts and core ideas*. Washington, D.C.: The National Academies Press.

Nyman, S. J., Nafziger, M. A., & Smith, T. B. (2011). Client outcomes across counselor training level with a multi-tiered supervision model. *Journal of Counseling and Development*, *88*, 204–209.

Ogden, T. (1992). Projective identification and psychotherapeutic technique. New York: Jason Aronson.

Orlinsky, D., & Ronnstad, M. (2005). *How psychotherapists develop: Therapeutic work and professional development*. Washington, D.C.: American Psychological Association.

Paul, R. (2012). *Critical thinking: What every person needs to survive in a rapidly changing world*. Tomales, Calif.: Foundation for Critical Thinking Press.

Pressley, M., & McCormick, C. (1995). *Advanced educational psychology for educators, researchers and policymakers*. New York: HarperCollins College Publishers.

Prins, F., Veenman, M. & Elshout, J. (2006). The impact of intellectual ability and metacognition on learning: New support for the threshold of problematicity theory. *Learning and Instruction*, *16*(4), 374–387.

Prouty, G., Van Werde, D., & Pörtner, M. (2002). *Pre-therapy: Reaching contact impaired clients*. Monmouth, UK: PCCS Books.

Pugh, K. J., & Bergin, D. A. (2006). Motivational influences on transfer. *Educational Psychologist*, *41*(3), 147–160.

Racker, H. (1968). *Transference and countertransference*. New York: International Universities Press.

Raney, J. (1983). *Listening and interpreting: The challenge of the work of Robert Langs*. New York: Aronson.

Rittle-Johnson, B. (2019). Iterative development of conceptual and procedural knowledge in mathematics learning and instruction. In J. Dunlosky & K. Rawson (Eds.), *The Cambridge handbook of cognition and education* (pp. 124–147). Cambridge, UK: Cambridge University Press.

Rittle-Johnson, B., Siegler, R., & Alibali, M. (2001). Developing conceptual understanding and procedural skill in mathematics: An iterative process. *Journal of Educational Psychology*, *93*, 346–362.

Rousmaniere, T. (2016). *Deliberate practice for psychotherapists: A guide to improving clinical effectiveness*. New York: Routledge.

Rousmaniere, T. (2019). *Mastering the inner skills of psychotherapy: A deliberate practice manual*. Seattle, Wash.: Gold Lantern.

Rousmaniere, T., Goodyear, R., Miller, S., & Wampold, B. (Eds.). (2017). *The cycle of excellence: Using deliberate practice to improve supervision and training*. New York: Wiley.

Scheerens, J., & Bosker, R. J. (1997). *The foundations of educational effectiveness*. Oxford: Pergamon.

Schraw, G. (2006). Knowledge: Structures and processes. In P. Alexander, P. Winne, E. Anderman, & L. Como (Eds.), *Handbook of educational psychology* (pp. 245–263). New York: Routledge.

Shapiro, L., & Stoltz, S. (2019). Embodied cognition and its significance for education. *Theory and Research in Education*, 17(1), 19–39.

Smith, D. (2018). *Hidden conversations: An introduction to communicative psychoanalysis*. New York: Routledge.

Songer, N., & Kali, Y. (2022). Science education and the learning sciences: A co-evolutionary approach. In R. Sawyer (Ed.), *The Cambridge handbook of the learning sciences* (3rd ed., pp. 486–503). Cambridge, UK: Cambridge University Press.

Tansey, M., & Burke, W. (1995). *Understanding countertransference: From projective identification to empathy*. New York: Routledge.

Vardi, I. (2015). Becoming a "critical thinker." In M. Davies & R. Barnett (Eds.), *The Palgrave handbook of critical thinking in higher education* (pp. 197–212). New York: Palgrave MacMillan.

Varela, F. J., Thompson, E., & Rosch, E. (1991). *The embodied mind: Cognitive science and human experience*. Cambridge, Mass.: MIT Press.

Veenman, M., Prins, F., & Elshout, J. (2002). Initial inductive learning in a complex computer simulated environment: The role of metacognitive skills and intellectual ability. *Computers in Human Behavior*, 18, 327–341.

Wayne, D., Butter, J., Siddall, V., Fudala, M., Wade, L., Fienglass, J. GcGaghie, & W. (2006). Mastery learning of advanced cardiac life support skills by internal medicine residents using simulation technology and deliberate practice. *Journal of General Medicine*, 21(3), 251–256.

Chapter 7

Conditional Knowledge: When and Why We Use Our Skills

Jon Frederickson

Conditional knowledge is knowing *when* and *why* we use interventions and listening strategies (Flavell, 1979; Pintrich, Wolters, & Baxter, 2000; Schneider & Pressley, 1997). For students to transfer their learning to new and novel situations, they learn what to do. And they must also *understand* when and why to intervene—conditional knowledge. Then declarative, procedural, and conditional knowledge become integrated for effective transfer. For instance, a student might know an intervention but not when or why to use it. Used randomly, the intervention remains ineffective. "[P]rocedures learned without conceptual understanding tend to be error-prone, are easily forgotten, and do not transfer easily to novel problem types" (Ohlsson and Rees, 1991, p. 104).

Conditional knowledge can determine the outcome of therapy. When students don't know why and when to use a particular intervention, therapy becomes haphazard. And they will intervene without a clear purpose. All interventions have a time and place where they are helpful and where they are not. And they have a specific purpose. One might say students learn that every intervention works ... until it doesn't.

In all models of therapy, the therapist asks about the problem the patient wants help with. Next, the therapist and patient develop a consensus on the problem to work on and the goal to achieve. However, the therapist who keeps starting each session encourages passivity in the patient. Thus, an intervention that initially promoted an alliance eventually encourages a misalliance. By continually starting every session, the therapist takes away the patient's initiative.

A therapist may try to understand the patient using the concept of conflict but finds himself getting stuck. But he doesn't understand why. When the supervisor invites the student to examine the patient's level of engagement, the student realizes the patient is distant and uninvolved. Now, the therapist learns to use the concept of transference to analyze the quality of the relationship. And he learns conditional knowledge: when one concept for organizing clinical data does not work, look at the case from a

DOI: 10.4324/9781003488637-7

different point of view, using a different concept. As a result, rather than address only conflict, he can also address the ways in which the patient relates to him.

In these examples, we see how the therapist learns the conditions under which an intervention or a concept works and doesn't work. And he learns to change his interventions or clinical thinking strategies to fit the conditions. For therapy to be effective the therapist must know when and why an intervention is useful or not.

To teach the principles and clinical thinking that guide interventions, the teacher can ask the student to explain how she selected a particular intervention and why she used it (Chi et al., 1989). Metacognitive questions help students explain these features (Renkl & Eitel, 2019). Then students learn the principles guiding their interventions. As a result, those principles can guide their thinking when approaching new clinical problems with patients.

Metacognitive questions develop students' conditional knowledge. Ask students to explain their problem-solving using the principles and concepts they are learning. Explanations of their analyses, interventions, and problem-solving make them more successful as learners (Chi et al., 1989). Further, self-explanations improve their conceptual knowledge and problem-solving performance (Renkl & Eitel, 2019).

Answers based on principles help students transfer those principles to new problems (Schalk, Saalbach, & Stern, 2016). Now, problems correspond to an underlying principle, which can apply to new patients (Renkl & Eitel, 2019). They learn to see through the surface features (symptoms) and select the correct principles. Then, they see the relationships between principles, concepts, and patients.

At first, "highly structured prompts constrain and, therefore, help the learners to provide principle-based self-explanations" (Renkl & Eitel, 2019, p. 535). For example, ask students where the patient's response is on the triangle of conflict. Thereby, you teach a basic principle—always use a psychological concept to analyze the patient's response to intervention.

Table 7.1 Recommendations for fostering students' self-Explanations

Ask students to self-explain cases in a principle-based manner.
Use prompts to provide structure if students are not used to explaining the principles guiding their work.
Invite students to self-explain correct and incorrect solutions side by side. Then they can remember correct and incorrect knowledge and integrate it.
Fade out self-explaining requirements once they have understood a principle. Now, they can automatize the skill.
Assess the quality of the student's self-explanation.

Source: Adapted from Renkl & Eitel, 2019, p. 542.

When you ask students to analyze the latent content in a patient's statements, you teach another principle——consciously choose a listening approach. Highly structured prompts help students learn the basic principles of psychotherapy.

It is impossible to describe conditional knowledge as it applies to all interventions. However, let us illustrate conditional knowledge for listening strategies used in psychotherapy.

Listening to manifest content

We always listen to manifest content. The literal meaning of the patient's words shows how the patient understands her problems. Laypersons listen this way habitually. Therapists use this approach intentionally to engage in two kinds of reflection. We may engage in static reflection——reflecting what the patient said without adding anything. Or we may offer a dynamic reflection——reflecting what the patient said while highlighting an implicit desire for movement or change.

Conditional knowledge: when do we listen to manifest content? Always. Why? A conscious therapeutic alliance is based on the patient's conscious understanding of her problem and therapy. Therefore, we help the patient become aware of other elements, so that her conscious understanding of the alliance can expand.

Limitations: The patient can be aware of only what the defenses have not censored. And since they limit what she can see, they determine what she can understand. Thus, the manifest content is the product of unconscious defenses. For instance, an externalizing patient blames others for her difficulties. The defense of blaming directs her attention outward. So, she cannot look inward to see how defenses cause her suffering. "Others cause my suffering." This makes sense to her because the defense of blaming excludes any contradictory information.

Likewise, a patient who uses the defense of denial cannot see what she denies. Thus, her conscious understanding will lack the parts of reality her denial excludes. As a result, her story will make sense to anyone unaware of the information that denial leaves out. Thus, if the therapist listens only to the manifest content, she won't see what the defenses exclude. For instance, every clinician has experienced meeting a patient's spouse who is different from the patient's description.

The layperson may listen only to manifest content. However, the skilled clinician always listens from additional perspectives to discern the unconscious issues the manifest content hides. Since the manifest content is the product of defenses, it cannot reveal what defenses hide. For instance, denial prevents the patient from seeing what she does, which causes her suffering. However, if the therapist can help the patient see her denial, she can face the realities she denied. As a result, she will see the feelings, anxiety, and conflicts she didn't see. And she will see how denial determined what she could see. Thus, we always listen to the manifest content to understand the patient from her point of view. And we also listen from other perspectives to see what the patient's defenses do not allow her to see.

Principle: If the patient and therapist hear only the manifest content, they will be blinded by the patient's defenses that *create* the manifest content.

Listening to unconscious conflict in the conscious manifest content

We can also listen to unconscious conflict to help the patient see what causes her presenting problems. The patient describes a conflict with someone. Perhaps she describes a feeling. Or we can infer the feelings in that relationship. We listen to what makes her anxious. As we listen to examples of her difficulties, we can infer the feelings that relationships trigger. We can listen to what makes her anxious. And we learn how she avoids her feelings and conflicts. Thus, we can use her words to describe an unconscious conflict. For example, a therapist might say, "You mentioned you were angry with your husband over his affair. And then you said the affair was 'no big deal.' When you said the affair was no big deal, could that be a way to dismiss yourself and your feelings (*identifying an unconscious defense*)? And could that have prevented you from acting sooner (*identifying the symptom the defense causes*)?" "If I notice any self-dismissal occurring here, do I have your permission to point that out, so we can help you take yourself more seriously?" (*invitation to the therapeutic task*).

The therapist helps the patient see how a conscious behavior (saying "It's no big deal") has an unconscious function. It wards off and dismisses her feelings. Here, the therapist listens to the manifest content ("It's no big deal") and simultaneously listens to unconscious conflict (the function of that statement). The therapist who listens only to manifest content might believe it was no big deal. From the perspective of conditional knowledge, the therapist knows that listening from only one perspective will lead to failure. That is why the therapist listened to the function of the statement. As a result, she could see the unconscious defense of self-dismissal and infer how it could make the patient depressed.

Conditional knowledge: Patients often describe their problems and struggles in the manifest content. Thus, listening to conflict helps the therapist see what the patient does not see. We use this listening approach to form a therapeutic alliance. If the patient sees the unconscious conflicts causing her problems, she knows what to explore in therapy and why.

Limitations: Patients who externalize their responsibility onto others may object to this kind of listening and formulation. So, the therapist shifts to identifying and deactivating the defense of externalization. Some patients do not freely offer a problem they want to work on. These patients will require careful listening to latent content, conflict, enactment, and countertransference to understand the perceptions of the therapist that make them reluctant to share. Sometimes, anxiety disrupts patients' ability to describe their difficulties. Then, we regulate anxiety first before exploring other problems.

Listening for unconscious process in the manifest content

The therapist listens to the patient talk. However, suppose the patient shifts away from an anxiety-provoking topic. The therapist can analyze the process. "Does this shift help the patient elaborate on her desire? Or does this statement inhibit her?" In other words, shall we explore her desire or address her defense against expressing her wants? A shift in topics that inhibits the patient has a defensive function. So, the therapist intervenes. "I notice you are describing a thought about yourself, but a moment ago, you were freer to criticize your boss. I wonder what might have felt risky about describing your thoughts about your boss here?"

When the therapist helps the patient see shifts in her conscious thoughts that inhibit her, the patient learns to see how a shift might have an unconscious function. It inhibits her from elaborating on a forbidden thought, feeling, or desire. The therapist works only with the patient's conscious thoughts to stay close to her conscious experience.

Conditional knowledge: Why do we teach this mode of listening? First, it triggers very little anxiety in the student and patient. And it helps the patient observe how her mind unconsciously shifts away from dangerous feelings, thoughts, and impulses. As a result, she becomes aware of unconscious defenses causing her problems. Patients who see their unconscious patterns and how they cause suffering and symptoms will be more motivated to partner with their therapist to turn on those defensive patterns. Therefore, therapists who listen and help their patients observe unconscious defenses fortify the therapeutic alliance.

Limitations: This mode of listening may not help when patients are highly anxious or impulsive. Under these conditions, we regulate anxiety first. And listening this way may not work if the patient resists emotional closeness in the therapy or is projecting. Under those conditions, listening to latent content, enactment, and countertransference may be more helpful. Also, this cognitive approach may not help the patient experience the feelings that defenses ward off.

Listening for latent content

Here, the therapist listens to the symbolic meanings of manifest content. "How do the patient's words symbolize how she experiences the therapy?"

Conditional knowledge: When do we use this form of listening? Psychodynamic therapists always alternate between listening to the manifest and latent content to understand the patient on both conscious and unconscious levels. However, there are certain situations where we must listen this way. For example, consider an oppositional patient. We can listen to latent content to discern the unconscious perception of the therapist. For instance, if the therapist represents a tyrannical father, we understand why the patient resists collaborating. Sometimes, analysis of conflict or process leads to no change. In those conditions, we shift to listening to latent content to learn how the patient perceives the therapy and why the previous listening approach did not work.

Limitations: There are conditions under which it is not helpful to interpret latent content. It can be too experience-distant to help the patient. Bringing unconscious perceptions into awareness may trigger too much anxiety in fragile patients. Or making latent content conscious may reinforce the patient's projection. Listening from this perspective is always informative. However, how we use that information will vary depending on the patient.

Listening for unconscious enactment

Here, the therapist pays attention to the roles the therapist and patient may be enacting in therapy. For instance, if the patient is passive, the therapist may notice she is becoming more active. If the patient is quiet, the therapist becomes more talkative. Now, the therapist can see how she has participated in an interpersonal enactment. Seeing the enactment helps the therapist stop enacting her role. And as a result, feelings rise in the patient, and the alliance improves.

Conditional knowledge: When therapy is stuck, the therapist usually does something that keeps it stuck. Listening to the enactment can help the therapist see what she is doing. Next, she can see if this enactment occurs in the patient's other relationships. Listening this way can help when patients resist the therapy. When patients present with relational problems, listen for unconscious relational enactments in therapy.

Limitations: The first limitation is that the enactment is usually unconscious for the patient and therapist. The therapist can ask a supervisor or colleague to help her see the enactment she does not see. To fully understand the enactment, the therapist also listens to latent content and the countertransference.

Listening for unconscious countertransference

Here, the therapist pays attention to her feelings, thoughts, and actions. "I didn't feel this way with my ten o'clock patient. So why am I feeling this way now?" When the therapist can see her feelings, thoughts, and actions with a patient, she can analyze them. What role am I playing in the transference? Am I feeling what the patient felt with a parent? Or am I feeling what the parent felt? What function does this serve if I have these feelings and urges instead of the patient? Analysis of the countertransference helps the therapist understand the transference and the enactment in the therapy.

Conditional knowledge: Any time therapy is stuck, we may be keeping it stuck. In this condition, we pay attention to our thoughts, feelings, and impulses in the therapy we accepted but did not analyze. Then, analyzing our countertransference may help us see how we enacted a transference in therapy. As a result, we can analyze the transference rather than enact and reinforce the defense.

Limitations: Like enactments, the countertransference is usually unconscious to the therapist. In this condition, the therapist can ask a supervisor who can perceive the countertransference feelings that the therapist cannot see. Further, there is a danger of valorizing feelings as the primary source of information. So, we listen to latent content, enactment, and conflict. Then, we can determine whether the countertransference hypothesis is consistent with data from other listening approaches (Tansey & Burke, 1995).

Other markers of unconscious confirmation include shifts in maturation of communication (Spotnitz, 2004), shifts from acting out to symbolic communication (Ekstein, 1966; Langs, 1989a, 1989b, 2003), and shifts in types of defense or conflict.

One sign that students lack conditional knowledge is the ritualistic adherence to rules. Students use rules when they don't understand the principles and clinical thinking guiding our interventions. For instance, a student may repeat an intervention even if the patient is not improving. Then, we can ask questions to develop the student's metacognition and conditional knowledge.

Teacher: "Let's look at three patients where we used that intervention. As we review those three cases we saw today, what do they share in common? What is the principle guiding this intervention in these three examples?"

Now, the student can think about his thinking and interventions. And he sees the pattern that connects: the principle. Without metacognition, the student will not be aware of conditional knowledge—when and why we use a specific intervention. He can think only about an intervention. He cannot look at a pattern of situations using that intervention to see the underlying principle guiding its use.

Another sign that students lack conditional knowledge is when they intervene chaotically or impulsively. Again, we can ask questions to develop the student's metacognition and conditional knowledge. Each time the student responds chaotically, do not refer to her intervention. Instead, invite her to assess the patient's response.

Supervisor: [*After a student's chaotic reaction.*] If we take the patient's last sentence, did she describe a problem to work on, become anxious in her body, or did she shift topics?

Student: She shifted topics.

Supervisor: And when she shifted topics, was that the problem, anxiety in the body, or a defense against declaring a problem?

Student: A defense? [*The question reveals guessing rather than understanding.*]

Supervisor: You seem unsure. What is confusing to you? [*A metacognitive question to assess where the student is confused, so that we can help him.*]

After each patient response, the supervisor keeps asking where the patient is on the triangle of conflict. The student learns that interventions are based not on guesses in her mind but on assessments of the patient's response. She learns that when the patient declares a problem, she can explore it. When the patient's anxiety is too high, she can regulate it. When the patient uses a defense, she can address it and return to the focus on a problem.

Conditional knowledge shows therapists when, where, and why to apply their concepts and strategies. Then, they can use listening strategies and interventions at the right time for a specific purpose with the right patient. The teacher can ask questions to teach conditional knowledge:

- Why was listening to conflict helpful here?
- When would pointing out the patient's conflict be helpful?
- What did you learn about when to listen this way?
- Why did pointing out the triangle of conflict (Malan, 1979) help the patient form a better therapeutic alliance here?

Summary

Beginning therapists listen primarily to manifest content. However, when we listen in only one way, we become the prisoners of that strategy and the information it can yield. Therefore, instructors teach several listening strategies so that students can compare the information they generate to understand patients more deeply. Evaluation forms give us feedback after the session. However, analyzing each patient response allows us to get continuous supervision during the session.

Metacognitive Questions for the Teacher and Supervisor to Ask about Students

Conditional knowledge questions elicit reasons, timing, and context/situations for using concepts, skills, and interventions, answering questions "why" and "when."

- What metacognitive questions could you ask to help students think about when they would use an intervention and when they wouldn't?
- What metacognitive questions could you ask students so that they could explain which interventions they use with which patients?
- What metacognitive questions could you ask so that students describe the principles guiding their interventions?

References

Chi, M., Bassok, M., Lewis, M., Reimann, P., & Glaser, R. (1989). Self-explanation: How students study and use examples in learning to solve problems. *Cognitive Science, 13*, 145–182.

Ekstein, R. (1966). *Children of time and space, action, and impulse: Clinical studies of the treatment of severely disturbed children.* New York: Appleton Century Crofts.

Flavell, J. H. (1979). Metacognition and cognitive monitoring: A new area of cognitive-development inquiry. *American Psychologist, 34* (10), 906–911. https://doi.org/10.1037/0003-066X.34.10.906

Langs, R. (1989a). *The technique of psychoanalytic psychotherapy: Vol. 1. Initial contact: Theoretical framework: Understanding the patient's communications: The therapist's interventions.* New York: Aronson.

Langs, R. (1989b). *The technique of psychoanalytic psychotherapy: Vol. 2. Responses to interventions: Patient-therapist relationship: Phases of psychotherapy.* New York: Aronson.

Langs, R. (2003). *Fundamentals of adaptive psychotherapy and counseling: An introduction to theory and practice.* New York: Palgrave.

Malan, D. (1979). *Individual psychotherapy and the science of psychodynamics* (2nd ed.). London: Butterworth-Heineman.

Ohlsson, S., & Rees, E. (1991). The function of conceptual understanding in the learning of arithmetic procedures. *Cognition and Instruction, 8*, 103–179.

Pintrich, P., Wolters, C., & Baxter, G. (2000). Assessing metacognition and self-regulated learning. In G. Schraw & J. Impara (Eds.), *Issues in the measurement of cognition* (pp. 43–97). Lincoln, Neb.: Buros Center for Testing.

Renkl, A., & Eitel, A. (2019). Self-explaining: Learning about principles and their application. In J. Dunlosky & K. Rawson (Eds.), *The Cambridge handbook of cognition and education* (pp. 528–549). Cambridge, UK: Cambridge University Press.

Schalk, L., Saalbach, H., & Stern, E. (2016). Approaches to foster transfer of formal principles: Which route to take? *PLoS ONE, 11*. https://doi.org/10.1371/journal.pone.0148787

Schneider, M., & Pressley, W. (1997). *Memory development between 2 and 20.* New York: Springer-Verlag.

Spotnitz, H. (2004). *Modern psychoanalysis of the schizophrenic patient: Theory of the technique* (2nd ed.). New York: YBK Publishers.

Tansey, M., & Burke, W. (1995). *Understanding countertransference: From projective identification to empathy.* New York: Routledge.

Chapter 8

Metacognitive Knowledge: What We Learn by Thinking About Our Clinical Thinking

Jon Frederickson

Promoting Metacognition in Therapists

Metacognitive questions invite students to think about their thinking so that they can improve it. For example, when we invite the student to think about her thinking, we learn what she sees and doesn't see. What kind of thinking can she do and not do? What listening skills does she have or lack? Then, we know what to teach and which decision trees to use to teach that concept or skill.

In the chapter on unlearning biases and assumptions, we saw how metacognitive questions help teachers discern misconceptions driving the student's work. Then, the instructor can use decision tree questions to help the student become aware of those assumptions. And role-plays can help students experience the limitations of their biases.

When we teach declarative knowledge, metacognitive questions help students integrate new psychological concepts into old knowledge. These psychological concepts either replace or modify previous folk concepts. As a result, the student learns to think about the differences between her folk concepts and psychological concepts. And she can think about how they determine what she can see and think about.

Instead of unconsciously using folk concepts, students learn to consciously choose psychological concepts for clinical thinking. For example, they can analyze different patterns that cause symptoms and presenting problems rather than use only agentic, linear causality. During these shifts, teachers use metacognitive questions to help students assess their process of conceptual change.

- "What have you learned?"
- "How does this new information change your old knowledge?"
- "How does this concept change your understanding of the patient's difficulties?"

DOI: 10.4324/9781003488637-8

- "What does this concept allow you to see that you didn't see before?"
- "How does this concept change how you can listen to the patient?"
- "How does listening to conflict change your former way of listening?"

These questions ensure that students integrate new knowledge so that their clinical thinking will change. Continuous metacognitive questions also allow the teacher or supervisor to monitor how students' thinking is changing.

We also use critical thinking questions to assess students' skills in procedural knowledge. How is the student integrating new skills into her work? How is she integrating her clinical thinking with her interventions?

Perhaps most importantly, metacognitive questions help students assess whether their interventions helped. Can the student learn from the patient's responses to change her thinking and interventions?

- "Did the patient's response validate your hypothesis?"
- "If not, how did the patient's feedback change your thinking?"
- "What are you learning from the patient?"
- "How did the patient's feedback change your old understanding?"
- "How did you change your hypothesis?"
- "How might you change your intervention?"

Metacognitive questions also help students understand the principles guiding our interventions—conditional knowledge—when and why we use specific clinical thinking and intervention skills.

- "Listening to the latent content allowed you to see that the patient viewed you as a potential killer. Based on that, why is listening to latent content important? When are good moments to shift gears and start listening to latent content?"
- "You saw that defenses are keeping the process stuck. Why is it important to formulate the patient's conflict when that happens?"

Metacognitive questions also help students make links between declarative and procedural knowledge.

- "Now that you understand the conflict the patient has presented, how might you describe to the patient his triangle of conflict (feelings, anxiety, defense) and show how his defenses are creating his presenting problem?"

Now, the student sees how clinical thinking leads directly to effective therapeutic action.

Metacognitive questions also help students integrate different levels of conceptualization to develop a synthetic understanding of a theory.

- "How do you understand your patient's statement from the perspective of *conflict*?"
- "If you analyze the *latent content*, how does that change your understanding of how she is relating to you?"
- "Now that you understand the unconscious *transference*, how might that help you understand the *countertransference* feelings you mentioned earlier?"

Metacognitive questions at successively higher levels of conceptualization help the student develop a more nuanced understanding of the patient. Further, she understands the levels of conceptualization within a theory and how they work together.

Thus, metacognitive questions help students make links between theory and practice and learn from the patient's responses. Only the student can make the links in her mind between different concepts, patients, and levels of conceptual thinking. Metacognitive questions help the student make those links. And responses to those questions tell the teacher what the student is integrating or not integrating.

Metacognitive knowledge is the glue that links all the forms of knowledge together. We teach declarative, procedural, and conditional knowledge. However, we use metacognitive questions to help students integrate those forms of knowledge. That process of integration transforms superficial knowledge into deep knowledge. Having described the multiple purposes of metacognitive questions, let us turn to our educational goal: deep knowledge.

Deep Knowledge

Learning facts and techniques is not enough. A deeper conceptual understanding helps students use their knowledge creatively. Without a deeper understanding of theory and technique, we see ritualism instead of creative interventions resulting from clinical thinking. Ritualism can take the form of habitually using the technique of reflection, a pattern we see in beginning therapists. Or students may habitually listen only to manifest content. Even the constant interpretation of transference in psychoanalysis can become a form of ritualism (Hoffman, 1998). So, how do we foster deep knowledge that leads to creative interventions based on a deeper understanding of the patient?

Connected learning: Each small piece of knowledge is linked to others in a network of related knowledge (diSessa, 2022; Sawyer, 2022). "Scientific expertise is organized into complex bundles of knowledge, not a simple list of isolated facts" (Sawyer, 2022, p. 3) As we saw earlier, concepts organize facts, and higher-level concepts order lower-order concepts into a comprehensive system of meaning-making that we call a theory. These concepts (e.g., defense, conflict, transference or, in CBT, maladaptive cognitions, response prevention, schema) are connected. Instructors teach students to make these connections to see how experts' knowledge is organized.

Focus on learning in addition to teaching: Instruction alone will not help students develop deeper conceptual understanding. Rather than focus on putting information in students, how can you help students integrate what they are learning? What experiences can you provide so that students actively participate in their learning? Which skill-building exercises, role-plays, and analyses of session videos would help students integrate their declarative and procedural knowledge?

Group learning: "Students often learn more effectively when they participate in collaborative activities with peers and the teacher, with the teacher guiding an improvisational knowledge-building process" (Sawyer, 2022, p. 3).

New knowledge builds on the student's prior knowledge: Students are not empty vessels. They come to class with a pre-existing folk psychology—preconceptions about psychological problems. While some preconceptions are partially correct, others prevent scientific, clinical thinking. If teaching does not engage their misconceptions, students will learn concepts to pass a test, but unconscious biases will continue to guide their work. Thus, teachers can help students see misconceptions and experience their limitations. Then, students can learn to use psychological concepts for clinical thinking. However, much practice will be necessary until misconceptions fade and psychological concepts guide clinical thinking (Pellegrino, 2022). Then, deep knowledge facilitates the transfer of knowledge and skills, enabling the student to create more effective interventions. Now, let us compare deep learning with traditional teaching practices.

High-quality clinical thinking occurs if students routinely:

1 Learn psychotherapy facts, concepts, and principles. *Declarative knowledge.*
2 Apply them to clinical problems. *Procedural knowledge.*
3 Evaluate their understanding, use, and mastery of those concepts and the therapeutic skills derived from them. *Conditional and metacognitive knowledge.*
4 Assess what they know and don't know so that they can direct their future learning. *Metacognitive knowledge.*

Table 8.1 Deep knowledge versus superficial learning

Learning knowledge deeply (findings from cognitive science)	Traditional classroom and supervision practices (instructionism)
Deep learning: Learners relate new ideas and concepts to previous knowledge and experience.	Learners treat course material as unrelated to what they already know.
Deep learning: Learners integrate their knowledge into interrelated conceptual systems.	Learners treat course material as disconnected bits of knowledge.
Deep knowledge: Learners look for patterns and underlying principles.	Learners memorize facts and carry out procedures without understanding how or why.
Deep learning: Learners evaluate new ideas and relate them to conclusions.	Learners have difficulty making sense of new ideas different from what they encountered in the textbook.
Deep learning: Learners understand the process of dialogue through which knowledge is created and critically examine an argument's logic.	Learners treat facts and procedures as static knowledge handed down from an all-knowing authority.
Deep learning: Learners reflect on their understanding and learning process.	Learners memorize without reflecting on their understanding or learning strategies.

Source: Sawyer, 2022, p. 5.

Through metacognition, students learn to think about the concepts they use. And they learn to think about how concepts, thoughts, and feelings influence their thinking (Ellerton, 2015). Thus, metacognition draws on cognition and informs it (Veenman, Van Hout-Wolters, & Afflerbach, 2006). Metacognition is central to clinical thought and expertise. So, let us examine the role of metacognitive skills in psychotherapy teaching and supervision.

> The capacity for metacognition is a profound predictor of learning (Wang, Haertel, & Walberg, 1990).

Assessment of the Student's Metacognition

To teach or supervise, the teacher assesses the most important thing for the student to learn today: the learning problem. To do so, the teacher asks questions to discern what the student sees and does not see. As she asks questions, she develops a theory of the student's mind. His responses reveal the concepts and assumptions he uses and the kinds of thinking he can and cannot do. She discovers the causal patterns he can see and cannot see. Finally, she assesses which concepts and skills he has and lacks.

Principle: The teacher asks metacognitive questions to develop a theory of the student's mind to guide her teaching and supervision.

Metacognitive questions help the teacher develop and refine her theory of the student's mind. To do so, she will think critically about the student's thinking:

- What assumptions or concepts is the student using?
- What kinds of clinical thinking can he do and not do?
- What steps in clinical thinking does he skip?
- Does he listen habitually by reflection, or can he choose different listening strategies?
- Can he see only linear causality, or can he recognize other forms of causality?
- Can he analyze the patient's response to intervention?
- Can he change his hypothesis and intervention based on patient feedback?
- Which concept or skill would be the most important one to teach today?

The student's responses allow us to diagnose his learning problem (what he needs to learn today) and problems about learning (attitudes or emotional responses that interfere with learning). Students' responses also reveal their ability to engage in metacognition.

To illustrate this process of assessment, imagine two students who present patients they are working with. The first student, Dick, says he was unhappy with the session. He read his notes from supervision the previous week and tried to apply what he had learned.

Student: I did what you told me to. But she kept avoiding the topic she wanted to work on. What should I do? [*Learning problem. The student assumes that the teacher can answer a clinical question without analyzing the data. He asks the teacher to give an answer rather than teach him how to think clinically so that he would know how to intervene.*]

Teacher: Well, let's look at the video of the session and see if we can understand what is going on. [*Inviting the student to engage in the first step of clinical thinking: look at the data so that we can use concepts to analyze it.*]

Student: But what should I do? [*Rather than engage in the educational task, the student presents his learning problem. He does not realize that we first look at the data to analyze it, generate a hypothesis, and then intervene to test that hypothesis.*]

Teacher: You're asking exactly the right question. And to know what to do, we try to understand the patient's response. Let's look at the video and assess each response. Then, with that information, we can figure out what to do. [*Inviting the student to engage in the task: assess each patient response to think clinically about the patient.*]

Dick makes a simple request which he assumes has a simple answer. He does not think about his assumption: "You can know what to do without understanding the patient first." Given his assumption, he does not think about his question, his thinking, or even the patient.

Now, let's shift to Dick's classmate Jane. Jane presented her case by saying, "I tried to do what you recommended. But I was confused when the patient kept trying to change topics rather than focus on her problem."

Teacher: How did you deal with your confusion?

Student: I looked back in the supervision notes and saw that changing topics was a defense. She was avoiding feelings over a recent separation from her husband. But when I thought of maintaining the focus, I was afraid I would be controlling the patient. [*A learning problem arises. However, she can think about her focus and her interventions. She is already engaging in metacognition.*]

Teacher: Is the patient consciously controlling the session's focus? Or are her defenses unconsciously controlling the focus? [*Inviting the student to link her idea of control to the function of defenses.*]

Student: Got it. Right. Her defenses are controlling the focus.

Teacher: Let's take your thought, "I'm controlling the patient." Where would that be on your personal triangle of conflict—feeling, anxiety, or defense? [*Inviting the student to think about and analyze her thought.*]

Student: That's a thought. So that would be a defense? [*She can think about her thinking and analyze it.*]

Teacher: Exactly. And could that defense inhibit you from maintaining a focus with the patient?" [*Inviting the student to think about how her defense affects her ability to engage in the therapeutic task.*]

Student: Wow! Like both of us could avoid a therapeutic focus. [*An insight based on metacognition.*]

Teacher: How about that!

Dick and Jane approach learning very differently. Dick cannot think about his thinking yet. Since he has no strategy for resolving his questions, he asks the teacher for answers. So, we teach him how to engage in clinical thinking. Jane can identify where she is confused and work on that area. As a result, the teacher can help her think about her thinking and defense. Dick and Jane reveal different capacities for metacognition. And those capacities determine how the teacher intervenes.

It would be easy to assume that Dick is unsuited to be a therapist, not psychologically minded. Some teachers might assume he has a psychological problem: "He needs therapy." However, we fail to assess the student's *learning* problem if we pathologize it. In that form of reductionism, we reduce an educational problem to a psychological diagnosis. Instead, a teacher could help him engage in metacognition.

Dick could not analyze what he did or reflect on why he did it. He did what he *thought* the supervisor told him. Since he can't think clinically, he follows the thoughts of others. Hence, his strategy makes sense. Following orders can be a problem about learning (a problematic style of learning) (Ekstein & Wallerstein, 1972). But Dick's inability to think about his thinking is a learning problem.

Example one

Teacher: Did your patient respond with feeling, anxiety, or defense? [*Decision tree question. This question helps the student pay attention to the patient's responses and analyze them as a first step in clinical thinking.*]

Dick: Defense.

Teacher: And can he see the difference between his feelings and his defense? [*Teaching the student to think about how the patient thinks.*]

Dick: No. [*Now, the student understands the patient's problem. So, the teacher can teach the intervention.*]

Teacher: How might you help him see how the thought covers his feeling and then invite the feeling underneath? [*This intervention helps the student see how analyzing patient responses—clinical thinking— leads to effective interventions.*]

Of course, the experienced supervisor sees that this student is unaware of the transference, which leads the patient to hide his problem. However, we start first with the most basic steps of understanding and analysis. Later, we can help him think about conflict, and, still later, about transference.

Example two

Having helped the student begin to learn to think clinically, we can go to step two: helping him think about his thinking. Here, is an example later in the supervision.

Teacher: You thought this intervention would help. But it seems like your patient didn't like it. If his comments about his pushy golf instructor symbolize how he is experiencing you, how might he have experienced your interventions? [*Teaching the student how to listen to latent content—how to view the therapy from the patient's perspective.*]

Dick: That he thinks I'm pushy? [*He hears the latent content. But he does not see how his actions could contribute to the patient's perception.*]

Teacher: Did you ask what he felt, or did you tell him what you thought he felt? [*Question to help Dick think about the effect of his interventions.*]

Dick: I told him.

Teacher: And who is talking more: you or him? [*Question to help Dick think about the effect of his interventions.*]

Dick: Me.

Teacher: How might the patient perceive that as pushy? [*Question to help Dick decenter and think about therapy from the patient's point of view.*]

Dick: Hmm. He might feel I'm pushy if I tell him what he feels rather than ask him. [*He is beginning to think about the impact of his interventions, a first step in metacognition.*]

Teacher: How does this change your understanding of the patient? [*A metacognitive question to help the student think about his learning process.*]

Assess the strategies that students lack, then teach them through decision tree questions. Metacognitive questions teach students to think about their thinking and assess it. Thus, they develop metacognitive knowledge.

Principle: Ask metacognitive questions to teach students how to evaluate their work.

Ever since Socrates and Aristotle, writers have pointed out the importance of metacognition. The developmental psychologist John Flavell (1976, p. 232) defined metacognition as "one's knowledge concerning one's own cognitive processes or anything related to them ..." Suppose I see I have more trouble establishing a therapeutic focus than doing reflection. Or I realize I could double-check my assumption about a patient before assuming it is a fact. These are examples of metacognition.

Teaching declarative, procedural, and conditional knowledge helps students think about the patient (object level). In metacognition, we help students think about their thinking (meta-level) (Nelson, 1996). Once they appraise their knowledge of their thinking, they can monitor, manage, and control their thinking (Cross & Paris, 1988; Pintrich, 2002; Veenman, Van Hout-Wolters, & Afflerbach, 2006). This provides the executive control necessary for expert levels of thought and analysis (McCormick, 2003).

Most students have not learned to think about their thinking. Thus, we teach them metacognitive strategies and how, when, and why to use them. As a result, students learn how to deal with problems and what to do if they cannot (Ozturk, 2016). Unfortunately, research has shown that most teachers fail to teach metacognitive knowledge (Kerndl & Abersek, 2012; Lai, 2011; Veenman, Van Hout-Wolters, & Afflerbach, 2006). As a result, "Classes are too abstract to challenge deeply held beliefs or too superficial to foster deep understanding" (Feiman-Nemser, 2001, p. 1020).

Metacognitive questions help students reflect on their thought processes to improve them. First, encourage the student to think aloud by asking decision tree questions. When her thinking processes become explicit, she can observe, assess, and think about them. She can reflect *while* doing a task to change her thinking—reflection while acting (as opposed to reflecting *on* an action) (Barzilai & Zohar, 2016; Schon, 1983). When therapists reflect on a therapeutic task while doing it, their thinking, learning, and intervention skills improve more quickly.

Metacognitive knowledge involves three major components.

- *Metacognitive knowledge.* What do students know about their thinking? What do they know about the tasks and strategies they use to gain knowledge?
- *Metacognitive skills.* How do we control our cognition and learning through planning, monitoring, and evaluating it? (Davidson, Deuser, & Sternberg, 1994; Schraw & Moshman, 1995; Veenman, Van Hout-Wolters, & Afflerbach, 2006)
- *Metacognitive experiences.* Feelings and anxiety rise when we think about our thinking and see how we construct our knowledge. What do we feel when we realize our thinking was incorrect and then correct it? (Barzilai & Zohar, 2014, 2016; Efklides, 2006, 2008; Hofer & Pintrich, 1997) (Chapter 4 on positive disintegration describes how to work with metacognitive experiences.)

Now, we will examine strategies for teaching metacognitive skills that lead to metacognitive knowledge.

Metacognition about Declarative Knowledge: Learning to Think about One's Clinical Thinking

The student's metacognitive knowledge about declarative knowledge involves thinking about the concepts and listening skills she uses for clinical thinking. When therapists think about their thinking and intervention strategies, they can improve their effectiveness (Sosa, 2011) and performance (Dignath & Buttner, 2008), and they can manage their thinking and learning (Schraw, 1998). The metacognition literature emphasizes strategies that apply across domains. However, this chapter will focus on metacognitive skills and knowledge specific to psychotherapy. (See Moore, 2015, and McPeck, 1981, for a review of general versus domain-specific forms of metacognition.)

Metacognitive Strategy: Decision Tree Questions to Think about Clinical Thinking

We can ask decision tree questions to teach students how to think about their thinking:

1 What concepts did you use to understand your patient?
2 What is the patient's conflict we see in this segment of the video?
3 What defenses did he use?
4 How might those defenses cause his presenting problems and symptoms? What information would help us feel more confident about this hypothesis?
5 When you intervene, what hypothesis are you testing?
6 Is there a more reasonable hypothesis we could formulate based on what we know so far?
7 Based on the patient's response, how might you revise your thinking?
8 Since your understanding changed, how might you change your hypothesis?

Likewise, we can ask decision tree questions to teach students how to think about their thinking when doing behavioral analytic therapy:

1 What concepts did you use to understand your patient?
2 What is the chain behavior analysis that we see in this segment of the video?
3 What schema did he use?
4 How might that relational pattern cause his presenting problems and symptoms? What information would help us feel more confident about this hypothesis?
5 When you intervene, what hypothesis are you testing?

6 Is there a more reasonable hypothesis we could formulate based on what we know so far?
7 Based on the patient's response, how might you revise your thinking?
8 Since your understanding changed, how might you change your hypothesis?

Metacognition helps students connect facts, concepts, and thinking to action. Memorized facts have no relationship to one another without a system of meaning-making. It's as if they are lying in a pile scattered on the floor. Students use concepts to see patterns in facts to understand how they fit together, much like seeing the layout of a jigsaw puzzle. First, we can see small patterns. As we put them together, we see how they form a whole. Facts fit into a discernible pattern of meaning that makes sense of the patient's life.

Teachers use decision tree questions to help students reflect on their thinking and assessments. As students master these decision trees, the teacher's initial questions can cue the entire sequence of questions (the decision tree) that we use to understand a particular patient response (Zohar & Barzilai, 2013). Thus, students learn the metacognitive activities to use during learning. Decision tree questions also help students assess what causes their mistakes.

For instance, a student's therapy was stuck. The patient had visited a psychic after her mother died. The psychic claimed the patient's dead mother had spoken to her and said to tell the patient she was fine. Afterward, the patient suffered many symptoms and came to the therapist for help. The following exchange shows one way to help a student think clinically.

Teacher: When she suffered from grief over the loss of her mother, what did the psychic say?
Student: She told the patient her mother was fine. And anytime she saw an eagle, it was her mother coming by to say hello.
Teacher: Did the patient believe that?
Student: Yes.
Teacher: Where is that belief on the patient's triangle of conflict? [*Can the student think about a fact and understand its function?*]
Student: Her triangle of conflict?
Teacher: Yeah. When the patient believes her dead mother is a live eagle, where is that on her triangle of conflict? Is that a feeling, anxiety, or defense? [*Decision tree question.*]
Student: Defense.
Teacher: And what kind of defense? [*Can the student think about a defense and understand it? Decision tree question.*]

Student: Well, it seems like a thought about animals. [*The student cannot identify the defense the patient is using. Thus, she cannot know what to do.*]

Teacher: Yes. And when the patient believes an eagle is her dead mother, what kind of defense would we call that thought? [*Breaking down a question into a simpler one that the student can answer. Decision tree question.*]

Student: Oh. Denial.

Teacher: And when your patient used denial, how might that keep her stuck in therapy? [*Can the student think about causality: how defenses keep her patient stuck? Decision tree question.*]

Student: It would keep her from mourning the death of her mother.

Teacher: How does the denial change your understanding of the patient? [*Feedback-driven metacognitive question. Can the student reflect on her knowledge and how it has changed?*]

Student: Denial keeps her from mourning her mother's death. So therapy is stuck because we can't help her face her death.

Teacher: How might you help the patient with her denial so that the therapy can get unstuck?

Decision tree questions help students see when their thinking leads to ineffective interventions. Once they can analyze interventions that don't work, they can change.

Metacognitive Strategy: Feedback-Driven Metacognitive Questions

In the vignette above, the trainee did not see how the patient's denial prevented her from grieving her mother's death. Supposedly, her mother was not dead but visiting her in the form of an eagle. I asked the trainee where the patient's response was on the triangle of conflict. Each answer from the student gave feedback to inform the next question. Hence, these are feedback-driven metacognitive questions.

The student's answer tells you the question to ask to help her think about her thinking. Metacognitive questions help the student experience what she knows and does not know and what she can and cannot do. Further, metacognitive questions also help build and protect the supervisory relationship because the instructor does not tell trainees explicitly what they missed. Instead, they uncover their mistakes by answering decision tree questions. Now, they know what to learn and where to direct their learning (Jacoby, Bjork, & Kelley, 1993).

In the following example, a student does not understand why his interventions do not help.

Supervisor: Let's look at your intervention. You said, "How do you experience that anger toward your husband if we look under your sadness and depression?" If we look at that intervention, what was the last word?

Student: Depression.

Supervisor: Does the end of the intervention prime anger or depression? [*Helping the student think about causality. Decision tree question.*]

Student: I hadn't thought of it that way. [*The student's statement implies that a new level of understanding is emerging.*]

Supervisor: As you think of it that way, what do you understand now as you see that pattern in the intervention? [*Helping the student analyze his intervention's impact. "As you think about it that way, what do you understand now?" is a feedback-driven metacognitive question. The student's feedback "drives" our next metacognitive question.*]

Student: If I end interventions with depression, I'll prime depression.

Supervisor: Exactly. How might you turn your intervention around to prime feelings? [*Metacognitive question: can the student use new knowledge to change his intervention?*]

Student: I don't understand.

Supervisor: You invited feeling, then ended with the defense of depression. How could you change the intervention, so that it ends by inviting feeling? [*Feedback-driven metacognitive question: he didn't understand the previous question, so I broke it down to make it easier to answer.*]

Student: Oh. If we look under the depression, how do you experience this anger?

Supervisor: Good. If we prime depression, what part of the triangle of conflict are we priming? [*Teaching the student to think about interventions and causality.*] [*Feedback-driven metacognitive question: can the student think about and analyze his intervention?*]

Student: Defense.

Supervisor: Rather than ... [*Using a half-question.*]

Student: The anger she's been avoiding.

Each answer from the student provides feedback informing the teacher's next intervention. If the feedback reveals a learning problem, the teacher can ask decision tree questions to assess the problem and teach the student how to think clinically. In the example above, the student had trouble integrating new information. So, the teacher offered feedback-driven metacognitive questions to help the student integrate new information into his old knowledge. When he said, "I hadn't thought of it that way," the teacher asked a question to help him think of it "that way," that is, to engage in metacognition. At another point, the student said, "I don't understand." Feedback to the supervisor—the student did not know how to analyze his interventions. Thus, the teacher's following three interventions helped the student do that.

> *Principle*: Each student's response provides supervision to the supervisor, informing her next intervention.

Good feedback doesn't necessarily tell the student exactly what to do. For instance, I didn't tell the student she was priming defenses instead of feelings. Instead, my questions helped her analyze her intervention so that she could identify her mistake and correct it. Teach students how to analyze the effects of their interventions. They then know what to change in their work.

> *Principle*: Rather than analyze students' mistakes, teach students how to analyze their mistakes.

The teacher assesses each student's response: what does she see, and what does she not see? What metacognitive strategy would help her most now? What questions would help her learn this skill? The teacher's assessment determines how she will intervene. And when a supervisory strategy does not help, she can analyze the student's responses, re-assess the learning need, and revise the teaching strategy (Ozturk, 2017).

> *Principle*: Decision tree questions teach students how to think. Feedback-driven metacognitive questions assess how students are integrating what you teach.

Here's an example of a student doing cognitive/behavioral therapy. A student presented a patient who was enacting a passive schema. The supervisor listening to the case noticed that the student was addressing the patient's maladaptive cognitions, but she also was doing all the talking.

Supervisor: You are doing a wonderful job describing the patient's maladaptive cognitions. As you described her self-critical thoughts, did we hear the patient's response? [*Drawing the student's attention to a fact she ignored.*]

Therapist: She didn't say anything.

Supervisor: Good you noticed. Who is talking more here, her or you? [*Drawing the student's attention to the enactment.*]

Therapist: Me.

Supervisor: And if you talk a lot more than her, what kind of schema will you be supporting? [*Can she use the concept of schema to analyze the enactment?*]

Therapist: Supporting?

Supervisor: Yes. If you talk a lot more than her, what kind of schema, relational pattern, will you be supporting?

Therapist: You mean I'm more active? [*Through her question, she enacts the passive schema. So I do not answer her question, which would enact that schema. Instead, I restate the question so that she cannot take a passive position in supervision. This avoids enactment of the parallel process.*]

Supervisor: What do you think? As you look at this segment of the video, who is active and who is passive? [*Can she think about the enactment?*]

Therapist: I'm more active, and she's more passive.

Supervisor: And what kind of schema might your activity be supporting here?

Therapist: Oh. Her passive schema. [*Now she can see and analyze the enactment. As a result of this capacity for metacognition, her work will change.*]

Supervisor: How might you change your interventions, so you no longer support that schema?

Once the student generates a better strategy, the teacher can follow up with metacognitive questions to deepen the learning.

• What do you understand about enactment now that you didn't understand before?
• How does your understanding of enactment change how you think about your interventions?
• What is still unclear for you about enactment?
• What are you learning about how you can co-create the patient's schema?

Metacognitive Strategy—Encourage Students to Assess What They Know

The following questions offer metacognitive strategies that students can use to learn how to think about their evolving knowledge and learning.

- What do you know about x (content topic for that class)?
- How would you assess your understanding of it?
- What do you know now that you didn't know before studying the readings?
- What are you having trouble understanding?
- Given what we just learned, what do you believe? Why do you believe it? (Grotzer & Mittelfehldt, 2012)
- Given what we just learned, what do you not believe? Why do you not believe it? (Grotzer & Mittelfehldt, 2012)
- What other evidence would make you change your mind?

When students assess what they do and do not know, they learn where to direct their learning. Students' answers also help the instructor assess where to help them.

Metacognitive Strategy: Help Students Think about Their Thinking Strategies

When students think about the thinking strategies they use to arrive at their knowledge, they will choose better strategies (Zohar, 2012).

- How could we evaluate whether the patient's response supported the therapist's hypothesis?
- What evidence suggests that the patient's defenses cause her symptoms?
- How could the therapist change her approach based on evidence from the patient?
- When comparing these two hypotheses, which one does the evidence not support?
- Why does the evidence not support that hypothesis?

Metacognitive Strategy: Help Students Identify Where They Are Confused—the Muddiest Point

At the end of a class or supervision, ask where students are confused. Just because you were clear doesn't mean that students are. If they are still confused, find out what they find confusing. What steps in clinical thinking are they still unable to do? What links between concepts or between concepts and skills are still unclear? What confuses them about a new psychological concept? The following questions will help you see where to focus your teaching and supervision:

- What was most confusing about the material you read today?
- What was most puzzling about how the patient responded to your intervention?
- What are you having the most trouble integrating today?
- What was the hardest part of learning this listening skill?
- What still does not make sense about …?

The Muddiest Point is an active-learning strategy used in many disciplines (Angelo & Cross, 1993). Asking "What do you find most confusing?" allows the teacher to identify what students do not understand and need to integrate. Give students practice recognizing what they do not understand or cannot yet do. When students identify where they are confused and why, they know where to focus their studies. And the supervisor knows where to focus her supervision. These questions also help co-create a culture where we recognize that confusion is a normal part of learning new concepts and skills (Evangeline, 2016).

Metacognition about Procedural Knowledge

Metacognitive questions about procedural knowledge help students think about listening skills and interventions. Feedback-driven metacognitive questions help students think about their listening choices. They learn to analyze how listening perspectives influence what we can know and understand. For example, a student who habitually uses reflection cannot monitor her interventions. Thus, she has no control over what she thinks or how she intervenes. Metacognitive questions develop the student's meta-strategic knowledge:

- What do we learn from reflection, and what is different about the knowledge we gain by learning to listen for conflict?
- What knowledge did listening to latent content add that you didn't acquire by listening to the manifest content?
- How does this change your perspective on listening to manifest content?
- How does using multiple listening strategies change your view of yourself as a listener?
- How does clinical listening differ from the listening approach you used before?

- What information do these listening approaches glean?
- What did each perspective allow you to perceive? What did each perspective prevent you from perceiving that you saw from another perspective?
- What are their methods of verification? For instance, what confirms a hypothesis in listening for process (the sequence of associations [Chapter 2]) versus listening to latent content (the symbolic meanings of the patient's words)?
- How does reflection differ from describing the patient's conflict?
- What do you understand now about the patient, and what strategies did you use to construct and justify what you know? (Barzilai & Zohar, 2016)

When the student can think about and compare listening strategies, she can monitor her choice of intervention. And she can see how it influences what she can hear and, thus, what she can think about.

Metastrategic knowledge allows the student to think about the strategies she uses, why she uses them, and the results they yield. For instance, she can decide whether to use reflection or analysis of conflict to guide her listening. In addition, metastrategic knowledge allows the student to transfer her knowledge to other problems with other patients (Kuhn et al., 1995).

Principle: The student who can assess the effects, usefulness, strengths, and limitations of different listening approaches has critical thinking mastery (Ellerton, 2015).

Metacognition about Procedural Knowledge:
Thinking about the listening skills and interventions we use to gain knowledge. Thinking about the patient's responses to interventions and what we learn from them.

Metacognitive Strategies: Thinking about Skills

Skill-building exercises develop students' implicit understanding of concepts and skills. Metacognitive questions help students translate their implicit non-verbal experience into explicit verbal knowledge. As a result, they can integrate the new skills and knowledge they practiced. Invite them to think about their new knowledge.

- What [key concept or skill] did you learn in this skill-building exercise?
- What did you learn about [the key concept or skill] in this exercise?
- How did the skill-building exercise change your understanding of this concept?
- What was hard about that exercise? How do you understand that? How is this skill different from your previous approach to that problem?
- As the exercise became easier, how did your understanding change?

Metacognitive Strategies for Analyzing Patients' Responses to Intervention

"How did the patient's response change your thinking?" As soon as we ask this question, we invite the student to a relational epistemology (Ananda, Medin, & ojlehto, 2018; Thayer-Bacon, 1997). In supervision, the students' conscious and unconscious supervision changes the teacher's knowledge. In therapy, the patient's conscious and unconscious supervision changes the therapist's knowledge. This often shocks the student, who thinks she will be the source of information to the "empty vessel" known as the patient. Instead, we help her shift to a new epistemology where the patient is not her student but her teacher. The supervisor might ask:

- Did the patient's response to the intervention validate your hypothesis?
- If not, what supervision is the patient offering you?
- How does the patient's feedback change your clinical thinking?
- How did you change your hypothesis and intervention?
- What are you learning about how the patient unconsciously supervises you?

Students have trouble grasping the relational epistemology we use in psychotherapy (Norris & Phillips, 2012). The layperson can state a conclusion with confidence. However, the psychotherapist's intervention is not a conclusion but a hypothesis to test. The layperson feels confident because he does not compare his answer with the evidence. The skilled clinician, however, assesses whether his hypotheses fit the evidence. He also assesses whether the patient's response validated his hypothesis. Further, he integrates the patient's feedback to improve his thinking and interventions. Thus, he learns from the patient. When patients' responses change the therapist's thinking and interventions, he has begun to think clinically.

It is not enough that a patient agrees with the therapist. That could be compliance: a defense. Nor is symptom reduction enough. That could result from idealizing the therapist: another defense.

> *Principle*: Confirmation of a hypothesis cannot come only from conscious communications, which may result from defenses. Instead, confirmation of a hypothesis includes unconscious communications from the patient which are not subject to conscious suppression in addition to conscious communications, which may be subject to defense. (See Gill, 1983a, 1983b; Langs, 1989a, 1989b; Raney, 1984; Smith, 2018.)

Some writers have criticized psychotherapy as unscientific (cf. Cioffi, 1970; Grunbaum, 1985). After all, if we cannot verify or falsify a hypothesis, no genuine critical thinking can occur. Making stuff up is not clinical thinking. Thus, instructors teach students metacognitive strategies for evaluating their hypotheses.

Metacognitive Strategies from the Perspective of Unconscious Conflict and Causality

From the perspective of conflict, unconscious feelings in the patient trigger unconscious anxiety. Anxiety evokes unconscious defenses, which cause the patient's presenting problems and symptoms. The theory of unconscious causality allows us to make several predictions:

1 An intervention that triggers unconscious feelings will trigger unconscious anxiety in the body.
2 Unconscious anxiety in the body will evoke unconscious defenses.
3 Defenses block the rise of feelings and anxiety. Thus, feelings and anxiety rise if the therapist helps the patient see and let go of defenses.
4 But if defenses remain unaddressed, feelings and anxiety will drop while symptoms will rise in the patient.

Several other predictions follow:

1 If an intervention does not trigger feelings or unconscious anxiety, the therapist is not exploring a conflict-laden problem. Or syntonic defenses/resistance are blocking access to feelings.
2 If a patient says it is her will to explore a conflict-laden issue, and no anxiety rises, her agreement is a defense, for example, compliance. The reason? Facing what we fear triggers anxiety. Avoiding what we fear will not. Thus, no anxiety will appear if it is not the patient's will to explore what she avoids.
3 If a feeling does not trigger anxiety or defense, it is a defensive affect, which functions as a defense (Frederickson, 2013). Or the feeling is not connected to an unconscious conflict. Thus, no anxiety or defense rises.

Examples of Assessing Hypotheses from the Perspective of Unconscious Conflict

A student presented a case in class where the work was stuck, and he could not figure out why. "She has declared her will to do therapy. But when we start to explore, we get stuck." So, we examined the transcript.

Student: Is this the problem you would like us to work on?

Patient: Okay. [*No sigh*] If you think it's a good idea. [*Projection of will onto the therapist.*] [*Learning problem: the student has a hypothesis—the patient's will is online. However, he cannot assess the patient's unconscious responses to see whether they verify or falsify his hypothesis.*]

Teacher: When the patient said "Okay," did she sigh? [*Inviting the student to assess the patient's response according to the criterion of unconscious anxiety.*]

Student: No.

Teacher: Did her statement trigger any unconscious anxiety in the body? [*Inviting the student to assess the patient's response according to the criterion of unconscious anxiety.*]

Student: No.

Teacher: Then, would her "Okay" be her will or a defense against declaring her will? [*Inviting the student to assess the patient's response according to the criterion of unconscious anxiety.*]

Student: But she said, "Okay." [*Student sees the conscious statement. But he cannot assess whether the unconscious responses confirm his hypothesis that her will is online.*]

Teacher: Yes. Consciously, the patient said, "Okay." Did we see a rise of unconscious anxiety in the body? [*Inviting the student to assess the patient's response according to the criterion of unconscious anxiety.*]

Student: I see. Her statement did not trigger any unconscious anxiety.

Teacher: Right. The will to explore an anxiety-laden topic usually triggers anxiety. Since no anxiety rose, where would her response be on the triangle of conflict? [*Inviting the student to assess the patient's response according to the criteria of unconscious conflict.*]

Student: Defense?

Teacher: Yes. We have a conscious "yes" and an unconscious "no," the absence of unconscious anxiety. What defense would that be? [*Inviting the student to assess the patient's response according to the criterion of unconscious defense.*]

Student: Compliance.

Teacher: Right. So, when she says, "If *you* think it's a good idea," what is that defense? [*Inviting the student to assess the patient's response according to the criterion of unconscious defense.*]

Student: Projection.
Teacher: Projection of ... [*Half-question.*]
Student: Will.
Teacher: Fascinating, isn't it? Let's look again at her "okay." What two unconscious clues tell us that her conscious "yes" is an unconscious "no"? [*Inviting the student to assess his hypothesis using the patient's unconscious anxiety and defense responses.*]
Student: Her lack of unconscious anxiety and her unconscious defense of projection.
Teacher: If her "okay" was a yes on a conscious and unconscious level, what would we have seen? [*Metacognitive question: has new learning changed old knowledge about assessing hypotheses? Can he make a falsifiable hypothesis?*]
Student: If her "okay" were a "yes," she would have sighed. And the unconscious defense of projection would not have come up right away.

Conscious responses can result from unconscious defenses. Thus, we cannot rely only on them to verify hypotheses. Instead, we also assess unconscious feelings, unconscious anxiety in the body, and unconscious defenses. The patient is unaware of these responses that are not under her voluntary control. From this perspective, an accurate hypothesis will trigger unconscious feelings, anxiety, and defenses. An inaccurate hypothesis will not.

We can use unconscious responses to test our hypotheses. Unconscious feelings, anxiety, and defense mean that the intervention has mobilized unconscious conflicts. Their absence suggests that the intervention did not. Thus, after each intervention, we assess whether the patient's response confirms that hypothesis.

> *Principle:* If patients' conscious statements conflict with their unconscious responses, we follow the unconscious responses to revise and test our hypotheses.

In the following example, a student presented a depressed patient who was not improving in therapy. The student thought the patient needed to feel her grief more deeply. However, the patient's symptoms were worsening.

Teacher: The patient needs to feel more grief, you say. That's a plausible hypothesis. Let's see what happens in the video. [*Invite students to evaluate their hypotheses by comparing them to data on the videotape.*]

Student: The patient told me her former boyfriend had texted her and told her never to speak to his friends again. And he called her a bitch. I'd like for us to start there in the session.

Teacher: Okay.

Student: [*Plays the video of the session.*] That must have triggered some feelings.

Patient: I feel so sad. [*Cries.*] [*No anxiety.*] Maybe he is right. Maybe I am a bitch. [*Unconscious defense: self-attack.*] [*Sobbing.*]

Student: Let it out. Terrible grief. [*Learning problem: the student has a hypothesis. But she cannot assess the patient's unconscious responses, which do not confirm it.*]

Patient: [*Sobbing.*] I feel so depressed.

Teacher: Let's pause. Your hypothesis is that the patient needs to feel warded-off grief. Is that right?

Student: Yes.

Teacher: Now, if this is grief she needs to feel, what do we predict her response will be after feeling it? [*Inviting the student to use her hypothesis to make a prediction. Then, we can assess whether the patient's responses confirm or disconfirm it. Thus, we assess the patient's unconscious responses of anxiety and defense.*]

Student: What do you mean? [*Learning problem: the student does not realize that a hypothesis always makes a prediction. So, we help her compare the patient's response to her prediction to see if it confirms her hypothesis.*]

Teacher: If feeling grief leads to healing, how might we expect her to feel now?

Student: Oh, you mean like she should feel better?

Teacher: If you think these tears are healing, how would she feel afterward?

Student: I get it. Yeah, she should feel better. But she doesn't. [*Now, the student sees that the patient's responses do not confirm her hypothesis.*]

Teacher: Wonderful you see that. It was a plausible hypothesis. You tested it. And how did she feel as a result here?

Student: Depressed.

Teacher: Whatever this was, feeling it made her depressed. How might we reconsider that hypothesis? When she felt these tears, did unconscious anxiety rise in the body? [*Teaching the student to use the patient's unconscious responses to assess a hypothesis.*]

Student: I didn't see any.

Teacher: I didn't either. Did any unconscious defense come in to block her tears? [*If unconscious feelings and anxiety rise, an unconscious defense will rise to block the feeling. That did not happen. Thus, tears were a defensive affect caused by a defense: self-attack (Frederickson, 2013).*]

Student: Well, she did say maybe she was a bitch. [*The student sees the defense but not its effect on the patient, how it creates her symptoms.*]

Teacher: Yes. And did that unconscious defense block her tears, or did it make her cry even more? [*Teaching the student to assess the effect of the defense to refine her hypothesis.*]

Student: I hadn't thought of that. Yes, she started crying hard then. [*Now, the student sees that the depression and sadness resulted from a defense. It was not grief.*]

Teacher: When she called herself a bitch, what kind of defense would that be? [*Inviting the student to analyze the unconscious response of defense.*]

Student: Self-attack.

Teacher: And if self-attack made her cry even harder, would these tears be the underlying feeling she struggles with? Or could they be caused by the defense?

Student: Oh. So, the self-attack makes her sad. [*Now, he sees that the patient was suffering from a defensive affect caused by defenses.*]

Teacher: And what influence might the self-attack have on her depression? [*Inviting the student to see causality.*]

Student: It would make her depressed.

Teacher: And if we explore her sadness from the self-attack, what impact will that have on her depression? [*Inviting the student to view the impact of her interventions from the perspective of unconscious conflict.*]

Student: This is terrible! I've been making her depressed.

Teacher: All of us have made this mistake. [*Validate mistakes as a natural part of learning to help the student have more self-compassion.*] Let's see how we can turn that around. Her boyfriend called her a bitch, right?

Student: Right.

Teacher: If she calls herself a name, does that help her feel her feelings toward him? Or could she be protecting him by turning the feelings toward herself? [*Inviting the student to analyze the relational function of the defense.*]

Student: It's a way she protects him.

Teacher: To test that hypothesis, how could you invite her to look underneath the tears and see what feelings are coming up toward him?

Student: If we look under the tears and depression, could we look at the feelings toward him?

Teacher: Then, see if asking for feelings toward him triggers anxiety. And then, we can see if feeling more anger toward him reduces the amount of anger she turns toward herself. Those responses will validate our new hypothesis. [*Teaching the student what the hypothesis predicts and how to assess the patient's unconscious responses to it.*]

Principle: Never dismiss students' hypotheses. Instead, invite them to compare hypotheses with the patient's responses.

Metacognitive Strategies from the Perspective of Latent Content: The Patient's Unconscious Perception of the Therapy

Many authors hypothesize that the latent content reveals the patient's unconscious perception of the therapy (Gill, 1983a, 1983b; Langs, 1988a, 1988b; Raney, 1984; Smith, 2018). This perspective allows us to assess whether hypotheses are confirmed or disconfirmed. For instance, a therapist offered an interpretation to the patient, who nodded in agreement. A nod might suggest the patient confirmed the therapist's hypothesis. However, later, the patient said the following:

Patient: I've been thinking about my uncle recently. He's hard of hearing. I know he means well. But since his hearing is bad, he usually misunderstands what we say. So, we keep repeating ourselves until he finally gets it.

Latent content: I am thinking about you. You are deaf to the meaning I am trying to share. I know you mean well. But since your hearing is bad, you usually misunderstand what I say. I keep repeating myself until you finally get it.

This unconscious response from the patient would disconfirm the interpretation. While the patient's conscious nod would feel nice to the therapist, the unconscious supervision would be painful. No wonder unconscious feedback is hard to hear! Yet, patients constantly offer unconscious supervision to the therapist.

In another example, the therapist acknowledged a hurtful statement he had made to a patient and its painful impact. A few minutes later, the patient, seemingly out of nowhere, began talking about a fifth-grade teacher she had. Although it had been a struggle to learn the material, she said, "It was worth it." In the latent content, the patient referenced the struggle in therapy, and it was worth it. In other words, the therapist's admission helped heal the rupture.

The patient responds to interventions with conscious and unconscious material. The conscious material will consist of specific, concrete statements about other people, which can be easily visualized. These statements may appear discontinuous, a jump from what the patient previously discussed. These conscious descriptions of other people can unconsciously symbolize how the patient experienced the therapist's previous intervention (Gill, 1983a, 1983b; Langs, 1989a, 1989b, 2003; Raney, 1984; Smith, 2018). Thus, these comments provide unconscious validation or disconfirmation of hypotheses.

Psychoanalytic theory predicts that we will hear positive imagery of helpful people after helpful interventions. And negative imagery of unhelpful people will occur after unhelpful interventions. So, we analyze the patient's response to assess whether the hypothesis was verified or falsified (Langs, 1989a, 1989b; Raney, 1984; Smith, 2018). Now, let us turn to the thorny issue of validation in clinical thinking.

We cannot rely upon manifest content alone as a criterion for validation. The patient's agreement may be due to compliance or idealization (Fenichel, 1941; Freud, 1964). Moreover, the patient's improvement may not be proof of validation. Even that can result from suggestion (Freud, 1955). Nor is coherence in the therapist's explanation an adequate criterion since wrong answers can be internally coherent. "Coherence is a precondition for the truth of a proposition, but it does not vouchsafe it" (Smith, 2018, p. 141). Conspiracy theories, for instance, are internally consistent because they exclude the facts that do not fit. Likewise, a student's explanation of a case may be internally coherent because he does not see the data contradicting his idea.

To assess whether a hypothesis is true or not (Popper, 1959/2014), we use metacognitive strategies. Only then can we change our hypotheses to develop a more effective therapeutic strategy.

> *Principle*: The therapist learns metacognitive strategies to assess whether hypotheses were verified or falsified. Then, she will know whether to pursue her hypothesis, refine it, or change it to develop a more effective therapeutic strategy.

Metacognitive Self-Assessment by Teachers and Supervisors

To develop your metacognitive capacities as a teacher, ask yourself the following:

- What assumptions do I make about what students should know?
- What assumptions do I make when students don't understand a concept in class or supervision?

- To what extent do I have evidence for those assumptions? (Girash, 2014)
- Do I speculate about their emotional conflicts rather than assess their learning problems, problems about learning, or metacognitive deficits?
- Do I teach based on what I want to put out or what my students are taking in?
- Am I holding onto a clear educational focus in class, or do I let the class wander?
- What do I find confusing in the teaching process?
- Why do I make the instructional decisions I make? (Girash, 2014)
- Do I acknowledge my mistakes in front of students? Or do I offer an unrealistic view of myself as an expert who never makes mistakes?
- Do I welcome mistakes as learning opportunities? Or do I judge students for making mistakes and get irritated with them?
- What do I know about teaching and supervision? (Girash, 2014)
- What would I like to learn about teaching and supervision? (Girash, 2014)
- What do I find confusing about my students' learning process?
- When student feedback annoys me, what perspectives do I use to understand that feedback?
- Am I telling or teaching?
- Am I doing the clinical thinking? Or am I asking questions, so that students do the clinical thinking?
- Am I asking questions to get the "right" answer? Or am I asking questions to discover where to help the student integrate new knowledge?
- Am I frustrated with students' answers? Or am I grateful for the supervision they offer me?

Summary

Students acquire a large knowledge base (Alexander, 2003). To build that base, offer feedback-driven metacognitive questions to help students integrate declarative, procedural, and conditional knowledge into a conceptual network (Bransford, Brown, & Cocking, 2000; Pintrich, 2002). Now students can connect facts, concepts, and interventions within an interconnected knowledge base.

Feedback-Driven Metacognition for a Learning Problem and Countertransference

We have examined a number of short vignettes to illustrate principles of teaching and supervision. Now, we will study a lengthier supervision transcript to illustrate how the student's learning process unfolds over time.

The process will show how to use metacognitive questions to teach a student how to assess interventions, patient responses, and the countertransference driving his learning problem. And we will see how feedback-driven metacognitive questions help the student integrate different pieces of knowledge into a synthetic whole.

The student presented a patient, a retired soldier who recently made a suicidal gesture, taking a sleeping pill and a few glasses of wine. He was seen in a clinic funded by the military. The patient has explored his feelings and suicidality to a degree with the therapist. And the patient turned anger onto himself and submitted to authorities. However, the therapist feels stuck. At the end of the previous session, the patient said he didn't want to come to the session because he would prefer to meet via video. The therapist said, "I felt like our connection has not been good." The therapist described a will battle. He wanted the patient to come to the office, and the patient wanted to do therapy on video instead.

Teacher: Is it possible this is a sign of progress? [*When a submissive patient no longer submits to the therapist, we see progress. Can the student see this? If not, why not?*]

Student: No, it's annoying. [*Learning problem: the student cannot see the progress in the patient. And he is taking the opposition personally: a problem about learning.*]

Teacher: Oh, annoying when the patient doesn't follow the will of the general, isn't it? [*A playful reference to the student, a former military officer, treating a patient at a lower rank.*]

Student: It is, yeah, that's a good point.

Teacher: It's very annoying when the patient doesn't follow orders. I agree. I should put him up for charges. [*A playful interaction to help the student shift from a fixed position.*]

Student: If I could only punish him anywhere near to the degree to which he punishes himself.

Teacher: Okay, so this is very interesting, isn't it? Could this be progress for him, that he can say no to you?

Student: Yeah. [*Here, the student submits to me. My question addresses progress, not the issues preventing the student from seeing it. Thus, we have a parallel process: the student submits to me as his patient submits to him.*]

Teacher: What's that like to realize this might be progress, that he can oppose you and say no to you?

Student: Well, I didn't think of it like that. So it's a bit of a relief. It feels like I don't have to do something with that.

Teacher: Well, could it be important to do something with it since this is an important piece of progress?

Student: Yeah.

Teacher: He's able to say no to someone. Yeah. He can say no to his therapist. And he's able to say no to a therapist in the military. Is that impressive for a fragile patient?

Student: I guess I didn't think about it like that. [*When a student says he didn't think about it like that, we can help him think along those lines. Hence, the feedback-driven metacognitive question that follows.*]

Teacher: If you think about it like that, how might the patient saying "no" to in-person meetings be progress?

Student: Uh, he can have some will. Huh? Yeah. Which is a big thing for him.

Teacher: Mm hmm.

Student: Given the context of the trauma he experienced,

Teacher: Because in a trauma, who gets to express their will? [*Inviting the student to think about the patient using the concept of enactment.*]

Student: The person who inflicts the trauma.

Teacher: The abuser. And who must have no will? [*Inviting the student to think about the patient using the concept of enactment.*]

Student: The victim.

Teacher: Right. Given that, how might this be progress that he opposed you and said no?

Student: That he doesn't have to succumb to my will around what to do in therapy. And he can, even though he's not kind of saying it in this way, and reflecting on it, he can enact it and feel more empowered.

Teacher: And might that even be a goal: the patient can say no to you?

Student: I think so. [*His understanding is still not clear. So I ask another question to assess where he is not clear.*]

Teacher: How does that change your understanding of the therapy process when a patient has a will problem? [*Metacognitive question: is the new knowledge changing his old knowledge?*]

Student: I think we should celebrate it, I guess? [*Old knowledge is not changing.*]

Teacher: You guess? [*A better question would have been: what is not clear for you?*]

Student: Well, no, I don't guess.

Teacher: How does that change your understanding of the therapy process? If his ability to say no to you is a goal? [*Metacognitive question: Even if his knowledge is not changing, the question will allow us to assess why it is not changing. Then we know what aspect of the learning problem to address.*]

Student: Well, it certainly makes me less frustrated with him. And it feels like I have to make him do (*slip of the tongue*), not make him do something. [*His slip of the tongue may reveal a wish to control the patient slightly out of his awareness.*]

Teacher: Exactly. To make him do something he doesn't want to do. How does that change your understanding of the therapy process if saying no to you is a goal? [*Feedback-driven metacognitive question.*]

Student: You mean beyond what I've said?

Teacher: Yeah.

Student: [*sigh*] [*The supervisee sighing (anxiety) is a sign that new knowledge is being integrated.*] I guess I'd want to hear more about how he wants to say no to me and about how wants to do what he wants to do.

Teacher: When he says no to you, is that a problem or a success?

Student: That's a success. [*My question unfortunately pulls for compliance (parallel process). So I ask a metacognitive question instead.*]

Teacher: And how does that change your understanding of the development of will in psychotherapy? [*Metacognitive question: is the new knowledge changing his old knowledge?*]

Student: I need a better lens through which to see something. I need to be able to differentiate what feels defiant versus what feels like progress. [*Now his learning problem is getting clearer because he can better differentiate healthy will from submission.*]

Teacher: Exactly. What may not be a problem may be very significant progress. Because if a patient has a habit of being submissive in relationships, what would we hope he'd eventually be able to do with you? [*Metacognitive question to help him differentiate defiance from self-assertion.*]

Student: Not be submissive, to be able to stand up.

Teacher: To not submit to you. How does that change your understanding of the work with him? [*Metacognitive question: is the new knowledge changing his old knowledge?*]

Student: I can't think of any. I mean, I can't think of anything other than.

Teacher: Because before you saw it, the goal was to get him to agree with you.

Student: Yeah, I probably wouldn't have put it in those words.

Teacher: He should agree to come into session to see me. That was your goal. Now, what do you understand might be a therapeutic goal? [*Metacognitive question: is the new knowledge changing his old knowledge?*]

Student: To not agree with me to not come in to continue to do things? [*He is still having trouble distinguishing defiance from differentiation—asserting his right to have a separate mind.*]

Teacher: To disagree with you. Insofar as he says no to you and disagrees with you, is that a defense against intimacy? Or is that the precondition to intimacy? [*Metacognitive question using the concept of conflict to help him differentiate will from defense.*]

Student: The second one. [*His understanding is still not clear.*]

Teacher: And what's that like to see? [*Metacognitive question: is the new knowledge changing his old knowledge?*]

Student: You know, it feels good. I felt like I wasn't getting anywhere. And I felt like we weren't moving forward. And one of my questions is, how do I get to move forward faster? [*He sees how a defense would hold therapy back, but he does not see the role of the patient's will in moving forward.*]

Teacher: But who moved forward? [*The patient, by declaring his will, moved forward. But the therapist interpreted this forward movement as the backward movement of resistance.*]

Student: He did. I did not.

Teacher: Exactly. So how might you move forward with this guy? Since he's moving forward, how could you move forward, so that the therapy moves forward? [*Feedback-driven metacognitive question.*]

Student: I need to move forward. [*His inability to answer more clearly suggests that the teacher's question was unclear.*]

Teacher: What might you do for the therapy to move forward? [*Feedback-driven metacognitive question.*]

Student: I guess, allow for disagreement, make space, and step out of the way of his will.

Teacher: To welcome a separate person in the room or the separate will.

Student: Huh. [*A moment of surprise may be a perfect moment to ask a metacognitive question.*]

Teacher: What's occurring to you? Something clicked. [*Metacognitive question: how is this new knowledge changing his old knowledge?*]

Student: [*sigh*] [*A sign of integration in the student.*] Just a deeper connection between what that looks like. I know on a head level the patient's will drives the therapy. That makes sense. But just how that's experienced and what form that takes is a different thing. My will won't mean anything if it's not really his will. [*His understanding of the concept of will is becoming more nuanced.*]

Teacher: And it's one thing to say yes to you. But it's another thing because when he says no to you, it's a yes to him.

Student: Yeah, I was going to say it's funny because I've used that phrasing with him before. [*He knew the concept, but it had no experiential content.*]

Teacher: But how are you experiencing this differently now, though, because you're getting this in some new way? [*Metacognitive question: how is the new knowledge changing his old knowledge?*]

Student: (*sigh*) I think it takes the pressure off me to make the patient do what the patient doesn't want to do and feeling not compelled to do that. And celebrate the opposite. [*Now, he sees more clearly how he pressured himself to make the patient do what he did not want to do. He is becoming aware of the countertransference that was driving his clinical decisions. As I keep asking to think about his learning, we will see learning problems or clues to the countertransference to address.*]

Teacher: What you thought was a problem you had to overcome is a success you can facilitate.

Student: Yeah.

Teacher: How is that changing your understanding of him and his will? And patients saying no? [*Feedback-driven metacognitive question.*]

Student: I think it changes my sense of what helpful therapy looks like, what the red carpet of therapy can look like, and how to roll that out. And how it can't be this setup of, "This is how we do it. So do it or go away!" [*He is more aware of his countertransference.*]

Teacher: Exactly. So very interesting. Isn't it? Working in a very nonmilitary way within the military? [*Linking the workplace to his enactment to see if he can reflect more on his countertransference.*]

Student: Yeah. And then obviously, these external pressures of "We don't know what to do with these patients, so fix them!" [*He can see the link between his countertransference and the institutional setting in which he works.*]

Teacher: Fix them! He's saying no to you. But he shouldn't be saying no in a military context. He's not following orders.

Student: Yeah.

Teacher: And they're saying he should follow orders. "He should be coming in to see me instead of doing it on video." [*An allusion to his attempt to dominate the patient.*]

Student: [*sigh*] [*The supervisee is recognizing his wish to dominate the patient.*]

Teacher: Shall we invite his anger at this point? Or shall we invite his will?

Student: I guess more will, right? [*His question indicates he is still unclear.*]

Teacher: Is this an advance in terms of expressing anger or an advance in declaring his will with you? [*A simpler decision tree question to help him differentiate progress from resistance.*]

Student: Declaring his will.

Teacher: Yep.

Student: I guess what's occurring to me is how much more space there needs to be for elaboration of the will. [*An increase in understanding.*]

Teacher: And what's the big word here we make space for?

Student: No.

Teacher: Yep. Because if there's no space for a no, there's no space for a real yes. A patient is not free to say yes unless he also has the freedom to say no to you.

Student: Right.

Teacher: And you remember when your little one was two years old? I mean, it was a no, no, no, no, no, no, no? And even now?

Student: She loves it.

Teacher: Truth be told, we all love no.

Student: We just don't like to hear it. [*More awareness of his countertransference.*]

Teacher: That's because people should always say, "Yes, sir. Whatever you want, sir." So there is helping a fragile patient acquire the ability to say no. There's the history of abuse where he's not supposed to say no. And he's working in a military setting where he should always say yes, even though he wants to say no. That military context you work in always casts a shadow on the work.

Student: It does.

Teacher: So, this guy said, "No, I don't want to come in person. I want to see you on video." Okay, how could we celebrate his no?

Student: How can we make sure you have a good connection AV wise so I can see you while you're at home? [*His focus is on the audiovisual technology, not the patient's will. So he still does not understand the importance of accepting the patient's separate will.*]

Teacher: Mmhmm. "Thank you for ignoring my No." [*Pointing out how the student left out the patient's conflict over saying "no."*]

Student: So, you want me to say what I would say to him? Or? [*He may be complying, or he may be confused by my rapid shift to a roleplay, so I clarify.*]

Teacher: Well, you might say, "Wow, this is big progress, letting yourself say no to me. What do you notice feeling as you give yourself this freedom to say no?" Then he'll get anxious because now his will is out in the open. Then you can start to work with it. "Notice how you become anxious as if it's dangerous to let yourself say no here to me. And yet we know this has been a major thing in your life. As if you're breaking your father's law to say no to anybody. And is that a law you'd like to break?" That would be a way to explore and celebrate this essential piece of progress with all your fragile patients. Since they have usually been traumatized, their ability to declare their will can be underdeveloped.

The fact this guy could say no to you is huge. And saying no to you, knowing you're a military officer of some sort, right?

Student: Well, not anymore. But yeah.

Teacher: But that's who you represent. You're working for the military. You're a superior officer. The shadow of your military rank was always there even if not talked about explicitly. This is a huge piece of growth. How is your understanding of working with him changing now? [*Metacognitive question: is the new knowledge changing his old knowledge?*]

Student: One. I need to spend more time acknowledging, celebrating his will to do what he wants to do. And not just say that but show him that I mean it too. [*Now he is aware that inviting the patient's will is not merely a technique but a genuine acceptance of the patient on a deeper level.*]

Teacher: And to mean it, to be glad someone can say no. In a way, the patient must have the freedom to resist before he can collaborate.

Student: Can you expand on that? [*His question indicates he does not understand that the patient must be free to resist before he can be free to collaborate.*]

Teacher: The patient must have the freedom to say no to you in order to say yes to you. If he has the freedom to resist you, he has the freedom to collaborate. Then we have genuine collaboration with a separate will and a separate mind, rather than compliance without the patient's will. [*A feedback-driven statement.*]

Student: Oh, this is so essential for me. [*A new understanding is occurring.*]

Teacher: Uh huh. What are you understanding now? [*Feedback-driven metacognitive question.*]

Student: Because compliance is obviously the problem. 98% of the people that come in my door are going to be overly compliant. And how and what I need to do and say when working with these folks is to make sure their will is online. And it's not a 20-second thing for many of these patients. It could be 20 minutes, two sessions. [*Now he understands that when he asks a question, he is not asking for an answer—he is developing a relationship.*]

Teacher: What are you understanding differently now as you as you see this difference between compliance and collaboration? And collaboration means a person with a separate will saying, "I'm going to join you, we're going to do this together." [*Feedback-driven metacognitive question: is the new knowledge changing his old knowledge?*]

Student: I think I've been duped by pseudo compliance because I really want pseudo will. [*A very big improvement in metacognition:*

the ability to think about his interventions and thinking. The
supervisee is also clearly seeing his countertransference when he
says "I really want pseudo will."]

Teacher: Pseudo will.

Student: Yeah, pseudo will. But it really was another form of compliance in a lot of cases or different times. [*He understands he was pulling for compliance. How deep is this knowledge being integrated? The next metacognitive question might help us find out.*]

Teacher: What's it like to realize that the more no you accept, the better collaboration you're going to get? [*Feedback-driven metacognitive question.*]

Student: I guess if I can, and I have to watch this again, you know, so it sinks in. But I think if I can accept that, it will help me feel more helpful and be more helpful and not get in the way of progress. I see things that look like they're problems. [*Now he sees how he gets in the way of progress by viewing the patient's will as a problem. To help him integrate this more deeply, I use the analogy of his parenting.*]

Teacher: When you accept your daughter's no, when you really accept it, how does she feel?

Student: You're assuming something, Jon. [*Joking.*] I think she feels good.

Teacher: Yeah, she does. Obviously, there are times where you accept her no, and sometimes you can't. I get it.

Student: Yes.

Teacher: But when you accept her no, she's happy.

Student: Yeah.

Teacher: Oh, I can be separate from daddy. I don't have to want the same things. Daddy accepts me when I'm not him. There's room for me. He loves me even when I don't want the same things he wants. Daddy loves me when I'm not him. Such important messages. This seems to stir something up. What is happening inside?

Student: There's a lot in there (*sigh*). It's going to be a minute before I can put words to that. [*Crying.*] [*An emotional knowing occurs, out of which an experiential cognitive knowledge will arise. This will make sense of his countertransference-based learning problem. I will not explore the feeling or his past because I would be moving beyond my role as a teacher and supervisor. I trust him to make the internal connections that will lead to change.*]

Teacher: Take your time. We need the time for a kind of internal emotional digestion before words come to mind. Take the time for whatever that is. Give yourself the time you need. [*Silence.*]

Student: [*He continues weeping for a minute.*] [*sigh*] It's sadness for my own experience. Guilt for being a lot like my own parents. [*He makes the link between his child, his parents, and the patient. I will not explore this link. We address his emotions only insofar as they drive his learning problem in the teaching situation.*]

Teacher: Guilty as charged. Join my club. [*By identifying with his mistake and his guilt, I join him and help him bear his guilt rather than avoid it through self-attack.*]

Student: I guess that's what was getting in the way. [*Now he sees that he identified with his parents' opposition to his separate will. This prevented him from accepting the patient's will in therapy.*]

Teacher: Yeah, I resemble that.

Student: [*sigh*] Yeah, I don't think I need to say more. I kind of know what this is. [*He does not have to explore his past in supervision. His emotional insight has dissolved his identification with his parents' defense of not accepting a no. Since he sees the defense, he is less likely to enact it and can more easily accept the patient's will.*]

Teacher: Okay. You don't have to tell us what that is. Let's ask another question directly related to work. How does this change your understanding of allowing the patient's separate will to drive the therapy? Because it's what we're learning here. It's not only about the patient's will. It's allowing the patient's separate will to drive the therapy. [*Metacognitive question. The focus is not on his parents or his past. The focus is on his emotional insight. How is it changing his understanding of his learning problem, his problem about learning, and the therapeutic task?*]

Student: [*sigh*] I have a better understanding of why that makes me angry and maybe why I resist it. Even though I don't know I'm resisting. It's just, why am I seeing that as a form of resistance? And even though I know this about the military, even though I don't want to be part of that messaging, I'm still part of that. It just changes the dynamic of what's permitted in therapy. Was there something else you were getting at, Jon? [*An unconscious indication that something more is coming up within him, hence the next question.*]

Teacher: No. How does this change your understanding of the therapy process? [*Feedback-driven metacognitive question.*]

Student: Yeah, it's [*sigh*] it really [*sigh*] helps me understand at a deeper level what I can do, what I can't do, what I can control. And I don't know why. Yeah, I'm not sure what else to say. [*The emotional insight is still not turned completely into words. But it is still operating and will continue to have its effect after the supervision.*]

Teacher: Yeah, and what is it you realize you can control and can't control? [*Feedback-driven metacognitive question.*]

Student: Well, I can't control other people.

Teacher: Uhuh.

Student: Yeah. And I can't control their yes, and I can't control their no. Well, I can certainly prevent the preconditions for other people being able to say yes if I try to steer things in this way.

Teacher: Mmhmm. And what impact does that have? There seems to be a deeper understanding of how you cannot steer a patient. [*Feedback-driven metacognitive question.*]

Student: [*sigh*] Yeah, I've felt my work has been slow at times. And I haven't progressed enough as a therapist. It was sort of like, "Well, what should I read? What skills do I need to work on?" And the connection to over-working to overcome this. I guess what I now know is a will issue in the patient. I was overworking to make up for the lack of the patient's will, or absorbing the patient's projection of will, or facilitating further projection of will or ... [*A great increase in understanding.*]

Teacher: I need to control the patient's will?

Student: Yeah.

Teacher: Mm hmm. Big job.

Student: Yeah.

Teacher: So obviously, your parents must have been able to control your will. [*Said with humor.*]

Student: Totally. Yeah.

Teacher: And successfully so, right?

Student: "Are you sure you want to be a psychologist and work with sad people for the rest of your life?" [*A statement his parents made to him.*]

Teacher: Mm hmm. "Would you be willing to swallow my doubt as a substitute for insight? Could I get you to doubt your will by swallowing my doubt and then we can have this closeness of mutual doubt?" [*Mirroring what they said to him, and what he, in effect, said to his patients by doubting their will.*]

Student: [*sigh*]

Teacher: "Don't listen to your will, listen to my doubt." This is a very big thing in therapy to think that I'm never going to doubt the patient's will.

Student: Can you say that in a different way? [*His question reveals that he does not quite understand his role as a therapist.*]

Teacher: It's very different to say, "I'm never going to doubt my patient's will like my parents doubted mine. I'm always going to listen to the patient's will. I'm going to be curious about their will. I'm going to be curious about their struggles in declaring their will. When they doubt their will, I'm going to point that out.

I'm not going to try to control their will like my parents tried to control mine, I'm not going to doubt their will like my parents doubted mine. I'm going to welcome their separate will. This is a place where they have a right to have whatever will they have because this is their life. It must be guided by their will. And I must honor their will because their will is an expression of their life force."

Student: [*sigh*]

Teacher: Very different promise, isn't it?

Student: Yeah.

Teacher: How is this changing your understanding of the therapy process and the environment you're trying to create for a separate mind and a separate will? [*Metacognitive question.*]

Student: It makes me realize [*sigh*] I can say all the right things. But if there isn't a solid foundation of [*sigh*] respect for the other person's will, even when it's not in line with therapy, when those two things, their goals, don't line up, I can see how overworking does not get those things better lined up. And that will not get things lined up. I'll just get more compliance. And be satisfied but not realizing that's not really will. [*Now his understanding has deepened considerably.*]

Teacher: If we have a secret agenda ("I want you to want what you don't want"), if we're secretly using skills to get them to do what we want, it's not going to work. And you're letting us know there's been this kind of underground wish to get the patient to doubt this wish to be on video: "You should want what I want and come to my office instead."

Student: Yeah.

Teacher: I'll tell you a phrase I found very helpful in my own supervision, "there must be a good reason for that." "He doesn't want to come to see me. I wonder what I might be doing that keeps this patient from wanting to come in to see me? What would be a good reason for this patient not to want to come in to see me?"

Student: Uh, well, he said later at the end of the session, "Okay, now I have to come clean. I'm feeling homicidal towards people on the post." [*The student makes a preconscious link to the patient's feelings driving the defense of missing sessions.*]

Teacher: Uh huh. And you're on the post? [*A link to see if the student can see this consciously.*]

Student: That's it. Yeah, we didn't make that link. [*He does now.*]

Teacher: Why would this guy be feeling homicidal? [*Inviting the student to think about the cause for the patient's defense of feeling homicidal.*]

Student: He cares about me, and because he doesn't want to kill me.

Teacher: But why would he feel homicidal urges towards you?

Student: Because I'm trying to make him do something he doesn't want to do. And in the way other people made him do things he didn't want to do. And I'm reenacting something traumatic. It makes sense he wants to kill somebody. [*Now he sees the link: rejecting the patient's will triggers anger. And the patient wards off his anger through suicidal and homicidal ideation.*]

Teacher: This looks like an easy thing to take care of.

Student: Well, now!

Teacher: How is this changing your understanding of why he doesn't want to come in? [*Metacognitive question to assess how the new learning is changing his old understanding of the patient.*]

Student: [*sigh*] Well, it's a will battle I cannot win. And I need to respect and acknowledge and celebrate his will, which will be very disarming for him because he'll be totally surprised. I think it will throw things back on kilter, not off-kilter.

Teacher: Right.

Student: Yeah, no wonder it's felt like I've been tiptoeing around him.

Teacher: Right. Because in a sense, what have you told him he shouldn't bring into your office? A no. Is it possible he is following your orders? [*A metacognitive question inviting the student to consider how his actions might reinforce the patient's "resistance."*]

Student: By staying home, yeah! So you're saying if I want them to come back in here, then I have to be curious about his no. [*"So you're saying" suggests that he is attributing his insight to me rather than integrating it within himself. Hence, the next metacognitive question.*]

Teacher: Well, if you want him to come to your office, how much of him do you want, what percentage of him, do you want to come into the office? [*Feedback-driven metacognitive question to deactivate his projection.*]

Student: 100%.

Teacher: Right. So if he experiences you want 100% of him, he'll have no trouble coming. But if we only want 50% of him, he's got to figure out, "How do I keep 50% of me out of that office, so I can make my therapist comfortable?" If you were seeing him in person, he'd have to come every other week to give you 50% of him. Or if he's on video, he can be 50% present. Patients are always trying to figure out, "How much of me can you tolerate? And how much of me will you kick out of this office?"

Student: It's funny you say that because in the last six weeks, there have been these reschedules, and he arrives a few minutes late, or he'll be on his phone in his car doing the video thing. Then he'll get a phone call, and then I'm sitting through 10 minutes of his phone call. [*Implicitly, he confirms my hypothesis. But, explicitly, he is not quite making the connection to his work. Hence, the next question.*]

Teacher: How do you understand that now? [*Metacognitive question: can he link his actions to the patient's responses?*]

Student: Now that he can bring 50% of himself, he's found a way.

Teacher: To protect you from the other 50%.

Student: Yeah. Fascinating.

Teacher: Yeah, what's coming together for you here? [*Feedback-driven metacognitive question.*]

Student: Just, [*sigh*] you know, I guess we all deal with fragile patients. But I think these are the ones that give the military a hard time because they flounder, especially if they experienced trauma in those first few years that sends everything into a tailspin. It occurs to me how they're defiant, and we react negatively to them when they refuse to do the trauma protocol.

Teacher: Let's think about it. If I wasn't open to your no, if I wasn't open to your frustration, if I wasn't open to your anger and complaints, how motivated would you be to be with me? [*A metacognitive question to develop the student's theory of the patient's mind.*]

Student: I would say I'm 100% motivated, but I wouldn't be. And then the first time any kind of feelings came up, I would bail on therapy.

Teacher: Sure. The more someone accepts us, the more motivated we are. And the less someone accepts us, the less motivated we are.

Student: Wait, say that again. [*His request suggests that he is having trouble integrating this new information.*]

Teacher: If I'm accepting the patient 50%, the patient's not going to be very motivated, right? Since I'm accepting only 50%, I'm not very motivated to meet him. Often, the patient's lack of motivation is a response to our lack of motivation to accept him as he is.

Student: Oh, my gosh, yeah.

Teacher: Oh, you're not the patient I want, so I'm not motivated. I'm waiting for my fantasy patient to show up.

Student: You know, it's so funny because my colleagues and I get all kinds of referrals like that. "I can't work with this person, they scare me or, or I don't know what to do with them." And these folks get bounced around. So they come with that expectation.

Teacher: Yeah. Someone says I'm scared of the patient, and I haven't met the patient yet. The only thing they fear is their projection.

Student: Right.

Teacher: And then projection becomes the basis of assessment. I must admit I've never been very motivated to meet any of my projections.

Student: Yeah, yeah, we meet them all the time.

Teacher: All right. Shall we go back to your video now?

Student: I don't know. This seems much more helpful than the video does. This growth in me will help me understand where and how I'm getting stuck with patients.

The student then talks about another patient whose symptoms had reduced by half. But now, when faced with a problem, she does not want to talk about it. And the student realizes he has become the engine for the therapy.

Student:	I've gotten stuck in a will battle with her. Whereas, previously, she wanted to look at this other stuff.
Teacher:	Shall we do a role-play?
Student:	Yeah, you want to be me, or do you want to be her?
Teacher:	I think I'll be the patient.
Student:	I thought you'd make it easier for me. [*He smiles.*]
Teacher as patient:	I know what I've got to face here, you know, with this assault and stuff, but you know. I don't feel ready to do that here.
Student as therapist:	Can you elaborate a little bit more on what ready would look like?
Teacher as patient:	Yeah, thank you for ignoring my unwillingness to look at that. I appreciate it when you ignore me. [*Helping the student see how he ignores the patient's conflict. We are working on the same learning problem but with a different patient.*]
Teacher:	Let me try it again.
Teacher as patient:	I know I really need to look at this, but I don't want to.
Student as therapist:	Okay. Yeah, it makes sense to not look.
Teacher as patient:	Thank you for ignoring my conflict there. Yeah, thank you. Thank you for addressing only one side there. Thank you. [*Helping the student see how he ignores the patient's conflict.*]
Student as therapist:	You want to look at it, but you don't know if you're ready to look at it. Now, what's it like to notice those two things at the same time?

Teacher as patient:	[*sigh*] Oh, you're addressing all of me, both sides of my conflict that triggers anxiety. [*sigh*] Yeah, because I mean, I know I'm not getting better. But then I know I need to look at this. But I'm wondering, if I'm not going to do it, why am I here?
Student as therapist:	Right. You're saying you're not wanting to look at it and you're coming in here? What's it like to notice that you're still here and yet you also don't want to look at this?
Teacher as patient:	Yeah, I mean, I just realized I'm wasting my time, you know, by not looking at it. But I don't want to look at it.
Student as therapist:	Right, you don't want to look at it and you're having a thought it could be a waste of time.
Teacher as patient:	Thank you for ignoring the fact that I come. [*Helping the student see how he ignores the patient's conflict.*]
Student as therapist:	Right, and yet you keep coming to therapy.
Teacher:	See, when we're angry, we forget the patient is in conflict, and we engage in our own kind of splitting. So this is very important. Even when the patient forgets he's in conflict we can remember he's still in conflict.
Teacher as patient:	It's just hard. I mean, you know, I remember the last time we faced this stuff, and it was hard.
Student as therapist:	Yeah, it's hard to face this stuff and yet you keep coming here.
Teacher as patient:	[*sigh*] Yeah. Um, I mean, I know I keep coming here, but I don't know. I don't want to go through that again.
Student as therapist:	Sure, I can understand. Yeah, you don't want to go through that and yet something about you keeps coming in here and talking about it.
Teacher as patient:	[*sigh*]
Teacher:	Okay, so what are you learning through the role-play? [*Metacognitive question: how is new learning changing his understanding?*]
Student:	How easy it is to get lost. I want you to want what I want. And a week ago or two sessions ago, you wanted this. It's a dumb 'aha' moment that you could want to talk about this then and be less willing to do it now. And it's certainly eye-opening. Like, oh, I thought I had will online. But it's not, it's dynamic. [*An essential insight: the patient's will to*

	engage in the task will vary from moment to moment, depending on the amount of anxiety that is aroused. Thus, a commitment from the patient is not static but dynamic, shifting according to changes in anxiety and defense.]
Teacher:	Let me give you a homely example. Let's suppose you're a weightlifter, and you could press 150 pounds. And let's suppose I put some extra weights, and it's 175. What's going to happen?
Student:	It's going to be harder to push.
Teacher:	You might not even be able to do it.
Student:	Yeah.
Teacher:	Well, you did 150 pounds last week. Right? We forget. Maybe it's a heavier emotional lift.
Student:	It's a good metaphor.
Teacher:	Right. We know, but we forget. But how much are they having to lift this time?
Student:	And to extend it. It's like, yeah, that other weight didn't crush me. I'm really concerned this is going to crush me. If I can't lift it, it will crush me literally.
Teacher:	Yeah, I have no right, of course, to ask you to lift anything you think might be too much for you.
Student:	There's a question I have. I'm trying to think of how to word that and how to know when it's a will issue versus addressing it as a positive goal. I guess it'd be like, is that something you'd like us to help you do? Is that something you'd like us help you build the capacity to be able to face this stuff? I guess that's where I'm getting stuck.
Teacher:	Do you want to play the patient now?
Student:	Yeah.
Teacher:	So, I'll be the therapist, and you'll be the patient.
Student as patient:	Okay. I don't know. I guess it's just hard.
Teacher as therapist:	I can see that.
Student as patient:	I mean, this is why I come in here. I feel so broken.
Teacher as therapist:	So you come in to do this hard thing. There's a sense you're broken. And wondering if you can do this hard thing. [*In the therapist role, I show how to describe the patient's conflict without taking sides in it. As the role-play continues, the student, in the patient role, will experience the impact of this principle of intervention.*]
Student as patient:	Yeah, I don't know what to do.

Teacher as therapist:	Yeah. There's this hard thing. And yeah, you don't know what to do. Whether to do a hard thing or not to do this hard thing.
Student as patient:	I mean, I know I should do it. Because that's why I'm having nightmares. But it's just hard.
Teacher as therapist:	And just because you should do it doesn't mean you have to. You could always do it later, or sometimes not even do it at all. No shoulds here. You have a right to wait as long as you would like to wait before looking at this.
Student as patient:	Well, you know, people at work want to know why I'm not at work, and I can't even tell them because then I have to think about this.
Teacher as therapist:	And there's no law that says you have to think about what's going on inside you.
Student as patient:	But I can't help it as I have to think about it.
Teacher as therapist:	Hmm.
Student as patient:	I mean, I want to get better. I want to get better. I don't know.
Teacher as therapist:	Yeah. Just because you want to get better doesn't mean you have to do that work right now. Maybe another, later time will feel better.
Student as patient:	I can't keep going on like this.
Teacher as therapist:	That's not true. People can go on this way for quite a while. You might be underestimating your ability for how long you can do this.
Student as patient:	Okay, I don't want to keep going on like this.
Teacher as therapist:	Yeah. You don't want to keep going on like this and find yourself going on like this. What's it like to notice that complexity inside you?
Student as patient:	It's hard.
Teacher as therapist:	Mm hmm, wanting to do this and not wanting to do this. Yeah. And noticing that hard complexity? And that real struggle inside.
Student as patient:	[*sigh*]
Teacher as therapist:	You know, a struggle inside you.
Student as patient:	I mean, I'm trying. I don't know what to do.
Teacher as therapist:	Yeah, yeah. Wanting to get better, not wanting to do anything, and noticing that struggle and not sure what to do with that struggle of wanting to get better, wanting to stay the same, and not sure what you want to do with that struggle inside you. And we may have to wait until you know.

Student as patient:	I mean, it's frustrating.
Teacher as therapist:	It must be very frustrating. I can appreciate that. Wanting to change, not wanting to do something. I can see how that struggle inside you could be very frustrating to you.
Student as patient:	But it's not that I don't want to. I can't.
Teacher as therapist:	Well, and if you can't, you can't. We have to accept that.
Student:	Can I interject something? I think in the last session I was getting hooked because I was ignoring the conflict or moving away from it. I was siding with only one side of the conflict. [*The student's shift out of role suggests that new learning has occurred. Due to the role-play, the student understands the principle of describing the conflict experientially and cognitively.*]
Teacher:	And describing his conflict in him, rather than "I have to take one side of this conflict and make him overcome the conflict." Right. You're describing, right? If he was riding the bike and falling all over the place, you couldn't ride the bike for him.
Student:	Yeah, if they weren't sure they wanted to get back on the bike, no amount of saying we can help you be a better bike rider would make a difference.
Teacher:	"Right now, your real struggle is: You want to ride the bike, and you don't want to get on the bike. Yeah. And can we notice that struggle inside you?" There's no struggle between you and the bike rider. "It must be frustrating because you want to learn to ride a bike and you don't get on it. That can be very frustrating to have the struggle inside yourself." Then he is frustrated by his defense. You're not frustrated because you're simply describing his struggle. Suppose we sat outside watching cars. And all we did was describe the cars going by: Mercedes, Ford, Chevy, Audi, Mercedes, etc. We wouldn't try to control the cars. We would describe them. That's your role here. You don't try to control where he drives or whether he drives. It's like a driving instructor in the passenger seat. "Wanting to go somewhere and your foot is on the brake. What's that like to notice the struggle you have about driving?" [*Using metaphor to make a*

	principle of therapy easier to understand.] What are you understanding differently about conflict? [*Metacognitive question: how is new knowledge changing his old knowledge?*]
Student:	About conflict?
Teacher:	Your position vis-à-vis the patient's conflict.
Student:	Well, I can't be a cheerleader and root for one side of the conflict in hopes I will bypass the resistance. [*Now, his understanding of conflict and resistance is much clearer.*]
Teacher:	"I want to pay attention to this side of you, and can we forget this other side? And next time when you come, could you leave that other side at home?"
Student:	I only want positive goals.
Teacher:	"Could you leave that other side at home? I don't want to treat the rest of your personality. So next time, could you leave it at home?" And the patient says, "Could we reschedule because I don't think I'm going to be able to leave that other part at home today. If that other part comes here, you're not going to be happy."
Student:	Part of the rules, Jon? There's no no, there's only a yes!
Teacher:	Only the proper part of the personality can come in rather than the whole kit and caboodle.
Student:	Yeah, that's all I want. Yeah. And I can see how it how I blind myself to being able to see that conflict and why I didn't get it. It's because of the different levels and ways I deceive myself into thinking I can make up the will and overcome the conflict by myself. [*Metacognition: now, he can think about his countertransference.*]
Teacher:	"If I ignore your no, I think I can bypass this problem."
Student:	Yeah. And if I focus only on positive goals enough and say them in a different way, I can get you to agree to do something you don't want to do. [*His ability to reflect on conflict and his previous enactment is much more nuanced now.*]
Teacher:	Yeah.
Student:	I don't know why that's a problem. I see very clearly why that's an issue. I can see why therapy goes slower for me than I feel like it could go.

Teacher: The more you accept into the room, the more the patient gets healed, and the faster it goes. And what is kept out of the room can't get healed. And then you get stuck because now I don't want that part, and the patient doesn't come back. But whatever comes in is what we treat. So the more we can accept everything, then everything gets healed. And then, we'll have an optimal tempo of healing.

Student: Wow, this, this was really helpful. Thank you.

Teacher: Yeah. So it sounds like something clicked for you. What do you understand now that you didn't understand before? [*Feedback-driven metacognitive question.*]

Student: You know, I had this sense in working with patients. I've felt like my work has been stuck. And in a way, for like the last six months ... there are impossible demands at work, and a boss engaged in splitting and projection and denial with me. These intense systemic pressures of being asked to do the impossible. And I can see how I've been trying to do the impossible. And that's coming out in my work with a lot of my patients.

Teacher: Do you know any therapists who have been able to do magic? [*Playfully addressing his defense: "I want omnipotent control over patients." And this defense was reinforced by his workplace which insisted on rapid, impossible results. The following responses are designed to help him let go of the defense of omnipotent control.*]

Student: There was a guy one time I thought could do magic. [*Smiles. A reference to me.*]

Teacher: Mmhm. And then you got to see his work. And then you realize: it's not magic. And some clinicians claim they get magical results. But that's where research is so useful because research shows nobody is achieving magic. We all want magic, but we've never seen it. We've never experienced magic. I saw a patient the other day for a consultation. He was hoping this would be magic. It's been very helpful, he said, but it wasn't magic. I can appreciate that. Because magic is that you could make some part of the patient go away.

Student: Make them better in three weeks or less.

Teacher: Right, and usually make them better by making some part of them disappear, so you don't even have to talk about it or deal with it.

Student: Providing more eloquent understanding of why they haven't gotten better. What a relief. Yeah, what a relief.

Teacher: Yeah, we're just a bunch of craftsmen. I've never seen magic, never experienced it.

Student: Yeah, I think I get impatient and ...

Teacher: And you know what impatience is?

Student: What?

Teacher: It's the refusal of what's here. When I'm impatient, I'm saying what is here shouldn't be here. I'm saying: even though the patient is this way, he shouldn't be the way he is. He should be this other way. "Could you quit being the way you are and be the patient I want?" These are very popular forms of impatience. But, basically, impatience is the rejection of reality. Patience is the ability to sit with what is without expecting it to be different than what is. And a lot of times with patients, we're not patient. We say, "Quit being the way you are even though I'm supposed to treat you for the way you are. Quit being borderline, although I'm supposed to treat you for borderline disorder. Quit projecting even though you come to me for help with your projection problem. These are all forms of I don't want to sit with what is. It's like I don't want to sit with the patient as they are. Impatience says, "Would you become the way you aren't. Then I wouldn't have to treat you."

Student: Yeah.

Teacher: I wouldn't have to face this reality of how you aren't. Who wants to face a patient who's so dismissive and contemptuous, like Debbie's patient? I mean, no one wakes up, nobody says, wow, I'd love to have that patient. People weren't saying, oh, I envy Debbie today. Nobody said that. Everyone's thinking, "God, I'm glad that's her patient and not mine. I hope he doesn't move down to Washington, D.C. or Halifax or I'd be screwed." But that's the patient we're having to treat. We wish it wasn't that way but that's what we have to treat.

Student: [*sigh*] Good supervision, thank you, Jon.

Teacher: How would you summarize what you've learned here today? [*Metacognitive question: how is new knowledge changing his old knowledge?*]

Student: I have to do, [*sigh*] it's hard to say in words. I need to make space for the patient's no and their ability to resist me to get true will online so it's not just mincing words. And I need to be open in dealing with my own frustrations and not using them as a vehicle to try to speed up the will process.

Teacher: Mm hm. And how's this experience changing your understanding of the role of will in psychotherapy? [*Feedback-driven metacognitive question.*]

Student: I knew it was essential. But realizing how essential it is in any therapy, the magnitude of what will is and what it means. And I think I understand when you say it's the engine of therapy. Now I know. I understand what that actually means.

Teacher: And what are you understanding now that you didn't understand before? [*Feedback-driven metacognitive question.*]

Student: That all the ways I've inadvertently tried to be the engine of therapy, even at 20% or 10%, in terms of the phrasing, or the speed with which I speak, or thinly veiled. "Let's do this thing because this is really what I want you to do, but it's really your goal." How superficial that can feel, especially with people who have sensitivities around issues of will. How there really can be no will from me. And how that will help me see more clearly and not pick up only on one side of the patient's struggle.

Teacher: When it was your will, you're picking up on that side.

Student: Yeah.

Teacher: And then when you get frustrated, you'd assume, well, he's just pure resistance. You would see one side or the other, and here we can we help him see both sides in him without importing one side over to you.

Student: Yeah, it's amazing, right? It's like how easy it's been for me to say, "This is about the patient's will," and see like it's not only the words they say; it's how deep that is for everyone.

Teacher: Right, and am I truly approaching him without desire?

Student: I don't think I have been.

Teacher: Without needing him to say or do or want anything?

Student: Yeah, I can't think of many patients for whom that has been entirely true, which is a bit humbling.

Teacher: But it gives you a sense of where your growth edge is.

Student: For sure.

Teacher: This is where you're working, to be able to meet the patient without a desire that they think or feel or say anything other than what they're thinking, feeling, or saying. Without a need for them to be any other way than how they are. No matter how pathological or crazy.

Student: Yeah.

Follow up from the student: *This last supervision you gave me has taken my work in such a positive direction. My pacing with all patients in sessions is slower, and I feel so much less like a used car salesperson, manically trying to get patients to "buy in" to treatment, an intervention, etc. I feel more like I embody the idea that I'm okay with the patient's will having to drive treatment, and that I cannot universally overcome will issues through ever-increasing levels of pressure. Along those lines, my work with patients' will in treatment has been smoother/calmer, and, as you've said* *before, it has made the therapy get snagged a lot less in those areas. This is very clearly related to the emotional insights/shifting I experienced and my capacity changing during my last supervision. There is more of a settled genuineness in my giving choice around "we can do this or not. Would you like to do this for your benefit so you can___?" type interventions.*

I've also had three sessions with the second patient we discussed last time. In the first session post-supervision, with this drop in my struggle with control, I supported his decision to continue with video therapy, validated his will and gave him praise for asserting himself with me, and apologized for pushing my agenda. He was deeply moved by all that and said that no one has ever apologized to him and meant it. In the next session, he let me know that he had been holding anger towards me ... for about a year and a half when my interventions had pushed him over threshold ... he left the sessions abruptly so he wouldn't act out aggressively. I thanked him for letting me know, validating and thanking him for the "gift" of his positive feelings toward me. We saw that he was holding incredible "guilt" for having abruptly left therapy because it was "disrespectful." I was able to own that I had disrespected him by not recognizing his limited capacity and had not listened to other ways [he] had communicated warnings to me due to being stuck in my own perseverating on [read "berating him"] with the question about feeling toward me. We processed how I needed to apologize for that, given it had made him worse. We looked at the enactment of him showing loving feelings by shielding me from what should have been and what is my own guilt for those actions. And we looked at how my limited abilities as a learning therapist contributed to that, and it's quite understandable he might be frustrated I hadn't been as helpful to him as either of us wanted.

I have other patient experiences too, but suffice to say, this past supervision was the most transformative to my own structure in helping me much more deftly (I have a sense of agility versus a previous sluggishness) navigate how/when to intervene with patients. I feel settled as a therapist in a way I haven't before, and I think patients really pick up on that.

Feedback-driven metacognitive questions allowed him to become aware of his enactment and countertransference. Often, a focus on the learning problem mobilizes feelings sufficiently so that the problem about learning emerges organically from the supervisee. Since it comes from him, he does not feel his boundaries have been violated. We are doing supervision, not therapy. Yet, by helping him with his problem about learning, our supervision had a therapeutic effect.

Finally, by following his language and cues, we discovered the internal cause of his enactment. Once he was aware of it, I did not explore his feelings further or his past. That is the task of his therapist not his teacher/supervisor. Instead, since he became aware of the enactment and the feelings it had warded off, I could feel sure that his work would change. Now able to face those feelings, he would not be as likely to use enactment as a defense against them. As a result, his therapy with the patient improved dramatically.

Summary

To foster metacognitive knowledge, ask students what they are learning and what is still confusing. Invite students to summarize what they have learned. Then they can integrate what they have learned and learn what they have not integrated. At the end of class, ask them how what they have learned has changed what they knew. If new information did not change what they knew, ask them why they think they did not change. "What concepts did you find difficult to understand today?" "What can you do before our next meeting to improve your understanding of those concepts?"

We can teach metacognition by instructing students in listening strategies. Then we show how, when, and where we use each listening strategy and its effects on what we can hear and understand. Next, students learn how to evaluate their clinical listening strategies and results (Veenman, Van Hout-Wolters, & Afflerbach, 2006). Finally, students can assess how to improve their listening strategy and performance (Baker & Brown, 1984).

Teach students how to think about the patient's responses, their interventions, and the thinking that led to them. Then, they can see what they have learned and not learned. And they can refine their interventions.

Feedback-driven metacognitive questions help the student integrate new knowledge so that genuine change occurs. Without metacognitive questions, integration stops, and the student's work does not improve. Hence, feedback-driven metacognitive questions ensure that teaching leads to genuine change.

"To teach intelligently, teachers should think metacognitively about instruction, so they effectively manage their teaching and use instructional techniques strategically" (Hartman, 2001a, 2001b, p. 168). Then students learn to think about their thinking, interventions, and patient responses.

Questions for Teachers and Supervisors to Ask about Students

- What metacognitive questions could you ask to help students explain the clinical thinking that led to their interventions?
- What metacognitive questions could you ask students about what they find confusing?
- What metacognitive questions could you ask to help students integrate patient feedback into their thinking and subsequent interventions?

References

Alexander, P. (2003). The development of expertise: The journey from acclimation to proficiency. *Educational Researcher, 32*, 10–14.

Ananda, M., Medin, D., & ojlehto, b. (2018). Conceptual change, relationship, and cultural epistemologies. In T. Amin & O. Levrini (Eds.), *Converging perspectives on conceptual change: Mapping the emerging paradigm in the learning sciences* (pp. 43–50). New York: Routledge.

Angelo, T. & Cross, P. (1993). *Classroom assessment techniques: A handbook for college teachers* (2nd ed.). New York: Jossey Bass.

Baker, L., & Brown, A. (1984). Metacognitive skills and reading. In P. Pearson, R. Barr, J. Kamil, & P. Rosenthal (Eds.), *Handbook of reading research, Vol. 1* (pp. 353–394). New York: Longman Press.

Barzilai, S., & Zohar, A. (2014). Reconsidering personal epistemology as metacognition: A multifaceted approach to the analysis of epistemic thinking. *Educational Psychologist, 49*(1), 13–35.

Barzilai, S., & Zohar, A. (2016). Epistemic (meta)cognition: Ways of thinking about knowledge and knowing. In J. A. Greene, W. A. Sandoval, & I. Bråten (Eds.), *Handbook of epistemic cognition* (pp. 409–424). New York: Routledge.

Bransford, J., Brown, A., & Cocking, R. (Eds.). (2000). *How people learn: Brain, mind, experience, and school.* Washington, D.C.: National Academies Press.

Cioffi, F. (1970). Freud and the idea of a pseudo-science. In R. Borger & F. Cioffi (Eds.), *Explanation in the behavioral sciences.* Cambridge, UK: Cambridge University Press.

Cross, D., & Paris, S. (1988). Developmental and instructional analyses of children's metacognition and reading comprehension. *Journal of Educational Psychology, 80*(2), 131–142.

Davidson, J., Deuser, R., & Sternberg, R. (1994). The role of metacognition in problem solving. In J. Metcalfe & A. Shimamura (Eds.), *Metacognition: Knowing about knowing* (pp. 207–226). Cambridge, Mass.: MIT Press.

Dignath, C., & Buttner, G. (2008). Components of self-regulated learning among students: A meta-analysis on intervention studies at primary and secondary level. *Metacognition and Learning, 3*, 231–264.

Efklides, A. (2006). Metacognition and affect: What can metacognitive experiences tell us about the learning process? *Educational Research Review, 1*, 3–14.

Efklides, A. (2008). Metacognition: Defining its facets and levels of functioning in relation to self-regulation and co-regulation. *European Psychologist, 13*(4), 277–287.

Ekstein, R., & Wallerstein, R. (1972). *The teaching and learning of psychotherapy* (2nd ed.). New York: International Universities Press.

Ellerton, P. (2015). Metacognition in critical thinking. In M. Davies & R. Barnett (Eds.), *The Palgrave handbook of critical thinking in higher education* (pp. 409–426). New York: Palgrave MacMillan.

Evangeline, C. (2016). Examining the effects of metacognitive skills on the performance of students. *Scholarly Research Journal for Humanity Science and English Literature, 3*(18), 4054–4058.

Feiman-Nesmer, S. (2001). From preparation to practice: Designing a continuum to strengthen and sustain teaching. *Teachers College Record, 103*(6), 1013–1055.

Fenichel, O. (1941). *Problems of psychoanalytic technique*. Albany, N.Y.: The Psychoanalytic Quarterly, Inc.

Flavell, H. H. (1976). Metacognitive aspects of problem solving. In L. Resnick (Ed.), *The Nature of Intelligence*, pp. 231–236. Hillsdale, N.J.: Erlbaum.

Frederickson, J. (2013). *Co-creating change: Effective dynamic therapy techniques*. Kansas City, Mo.: Seven Leaves Press.

Freud, S. (1964). Constructions in analysis. In J. Strachey (Ed. and Trans.), *The standard edition of the complete psychological works of Sigmund Freud, Vol. 23* (pp. 257–269). New York: W. W. Norton. (Original work published 1937)

Freud, S. (1955). Group analysis and the analysis of the ego. In J. Strachey (Ed. and Trans.), *The standard edition of the complete psychological works of Sigmund Freud, Vol. 18*. New York: W. W. Norton. (Original work published 1922)

Gill, M., & Hoffman, I. (1983a). *Analysis of transference, Vol. 1*. New York: International Universities Press.

Gill, M., & Hoffman, I. (1983b). *Analysis of transference, Vol. 2*. New York: International Universities Press.

Girash, J. (2014). Metacognition and instruction. In V. Benassi, C. Overson, & C. Hakal (Eds.), *Applying science of learning in education: Infusing psychological science into the curriculum* (pp. 152–168). Society for the Teaching of Psychology. http://teachpsych.org/ebooks/asle2014/index.php

Grotzer, T. & Mittelfehldt, S. (2012). The role of metacognition in students' understanding and transfer of explanatory structures in science. In A. Zohar & Y. Dori (Eds.), *Metacognition in science education: Trends in current research* (pp. 79–100). New York: Springer.

Grunbaum, A. (1985). *The foundations of psychoanalysis: A philosophical critique*. Berkeley: University of California Press.

Hartman, H. (2001a). Developing students' metacognitive knowledge and strategies. In H. Hartman (Ed.), *Metacognition in learning and instruction: Theory, research, and practice* (pp. 33–68). Dordrecht, Netherlands: Kluwer Academic Publishers.

Hartman, H. (2001b). Teaching metacognitively. In H. Hartman (Ed.), *Metacognition in learning and instruction: Theory, research, and practice* (pp. 149–169). Dordrecht, Netherlands: Kluwer Academic Publishers.

Hofer, B. K., & Pintrich, P. R. (1997). The development of epistemological theories: Beliefs about knowledge and knowing and their relation to learning. *Review of Educational Research, 67*(1), 88–140.

Hoffman, I. (1998). *Ritual and spontaneity in the psychoanalytic process: A dialectic-constructivist approach*. New York: Routledge.

Jacoby, L., Bjork, R., & Kelley, C. (1993). Illusions of comprehension and competence. In D. Druckman & R. Bjork (Eds.), *Learning, remembering, believing: Enhancing team and individual performance* (pp. 57–80). Washington, D.C.: National Academy Press.

Kerndl, K., & Abersek, M. (2012). Teachers' competence for developing reader's reception metacognition. *Problems of Education in the 21st Century, 46*, 52–71.

Kuhn, D., Garcia-Mila, M., Zohar, A., & Andersen, C. (1995). Strategies of knowledge acquisition. *Monographs of the Society for Research in Child Development, 60*(4), v–128.

Lai, E. (2011). Metacognition: A literature review. *Always Learning: Pearson Research Report 24*, 1–40.

Langs, R. (1989a). *The technique of psychoanalytic psychotherapy: Vol. 1. Initial contact: Theoretical framework: Understanding the patient's communications: The therapist's interventions.* New York: Aronson.

Langs, R. (1989b). *The technique of psychoanalytic psychotherapy: Vol. 2. Responses to interventions: Patient-therapist relationship: Phases of psychotherapy.* New York: Aronson.

McCormick, C. (2003). Metacognition and learning. In I. Weiner (Ed.), *Handbook of psychology* (pp. 79–100). New York: Wiley. https://doi.org/10.1002/0471264385.wei0705

McPeck, J. (1981). *Critical thinking and education.* New York: St. Martin's Press.

Moore, T. (2015). Disciplinarity and the teaching of critical thinking. In R. Wegeriff & J. Kaufman (Eds.), *The Routledge international handbook of research on teaching thinking* (pp. 243–253). New York: Routledge.

Nelson, T. (1996). Consciousness and metacognition. *American Psychologist, 52*, 102–116.

Norris, S. & Phillips, L. (2012). Reading science: How a naïve view of reading hinders so much else. In A. Zohar & Y. Dori (Eds.), *Metacognition in science education: Trends in current research* (pp. 37–56). New York: Springer.

Ozturk, N. (2016). An analysis of pre-service elementary teachers' understanding of metacognition and pedagogies of metacognition. *Journal of Teacher Education and Educators, 5*(1), 47–68.

Ozturk, N. (2017). Assessing metacognition: Theory and practices. *International Journal of Assessment Tools in Education, 4*(2), 134–148.

Pellegrino, J. W. (2022). A learning sciences perspective on the design and use of assessment in learning. In R. Sawyer (Ed.), *The Cambridge handbook of the learning sciences* (3rd ed.) (pp. 238–258). Cambridge, UK: Cambridge University Press.

Pintrich, P. (2002). The role of metacognitive knowledge in teaching, learning, and assessing. *Theory into Practice, 41*(4), 219–225.

Popper, K. (2014). *The logic of scientific discovery.* New York: Martino Fine Books. Original work published 1959.

Raney, J. (1984). *Listening and interpreting: The challenge of the work of Robert Langs.* New York: Aronson.

Sawyer, R. (Ed.). (2022). *The Cambridge handbook of the learning sciences* (3rd ed.). Cambridge, UK: Cambridge University Press.

Schon, D. (1983). *The reflective practitioner: How professionals think in action.* New York: Basic Books.

Schraw, G. (1998). Promoting general metacognitive awareness. *Instructional Science, 26*, 113–125.

Schraw, G., & Moshman, D. (1995). Metacognitive theories. *Educational Psychology Review, 7*(4), 351–371.

diSessa, A. (2022). A history of conceptual change research. In R. Sawyer (Ed.), *The Cambridge handbook of the learning sciences* (3rd ed.) (pp. 114–133). Cambridge, UK: Cambridge University Press.

Sosa, E. (2011). *Knowing full well.* Princeton, N.J.: Princeton University Press.

Smith, D. (2018). *Hidden conversations: An introduction to communicative psychoanalysis.* New York: Routledge.

Thayer-Bacon, B. (1997). The nurturing of a relational epistemology. *Educational Theory, 47*(2), 239–260.

Veenman, M., Van Hout-Wolters, B., & Afflerbach, P. (2006). Metacognition and learning: Conceptual and methodological considerations. *Metacognition and Learning, 1*(1), 3–14.

Wang, M., Haertel, G., & Walberg, H. (1990). What influences learning? A content analysis of review literature. *Journal of Educational Research, 84*(1), 30–43.

Zohar, A. (2012). Explicit teaching of metastrategic knowledge: Definitions, students' learning, and teachers' professional development. In A. Zohar & Y. Dori (Eds.), *Metacognition in science education: Trends in current research* (pp. 197–224). New York: Springer.

Zohar, A. & Barzilai, S. (2013). A review of research on metacognition in science education: Current and future directions. *Studies in Science Education, 49*(2), 121–169. doi:10.1080/03057267.2013.847261

Chapter 9

Conclusion

Jon Frederickson

Teaching Students How to Discover

This book has proposed a shift from a monological model of teaching content to a dialogical experiential model for teaching clinical thinking. Content is the "what" of teaching. But clinical thinking is the "why," the central skill that connects our knowledge, practice, theory, and personal growth. You cannot make those connections in the student's mind. However, your questions can help her make those connections.

Teachers who study the effects of their teaching "are the most influential in raising students' achievement" (Hattie, 2012, p. 24). Attend to what works and what doesn't work with students. With challenging and specific goals, students know what to work on.

Your questions reveal those goals. You do not merely put thoughts in students. Instead, you ask questions, drawing forth thinking from them. Their struggles with those questions teach them to think clinically. And your persistence demonstrates your faith in their potential. Ultimately, you teach yourself out of a job because you have accomplished your task. You have helped students learn from the true teacher—the patient. And you could do that because you accepted teaching and supervision from your true teacher—the students. But, in fact, we remain perpetual learners.

Just as the teacher or supervisor asks questions to foster a dialogue about learning, the students' responses provide both conscious and unconscious supervision about their learning needs. Thus, teachers learn by teaching and students teach us through their learning. And students learn to use concepts to engage in clinical thinking and to listen to the patient's depths. As a result, the training humanizes students, expanding their capacity for empathy as they discover "we are all much more simply human than otherwise" (Sullivan, 1940, p. 16).

DOI: 10.4324/9781003488637-9

References

Hattie, J. (2012). *Visible learning: A synthesis of over 800 meta-analyses relating to achievement*. London: Routledge.

Sullivan, H. S. (1940). *Conceptions of modern psychiatry*. New York: Norton.

Appendix A

A Transcript Designed for Deliberate Practice of a Listening Skill

The following study illustrates how you can use a transcript to create a test to assess students' ability to master a listening skill: in this case, listening to latent content.

Adherence Study: Listening to Latent Content

This study will test your ability to hear the unconscious, symbolic meaning of the patient's statements. You will be asked to discern how the patient's statements symbolize her unconscious perceptions of the therapy relationship. This is important because sometimes a patient consciously says "yes." But her unconscious response, represented by the stories she tells after her conscious response, gives us a completely different story. The stories she tells often reveal unconsciously what she is afraid to say out loud. When we can listen from multiple perspectives, we can gain a more complex and nuanced understanding of the patient.

T: So you have an appointment Monday? Your next psychiatry appointment?
P: Yeah, and I don't want to go. I don't know what the point of going is. What are we gonna talk about? I'm going to sit there. For an hour. Rocking. There's nothing to talk about with him. I really don't like my psychiatrist.

Put an X after the hypothesis that you think best fits the data in the latent content.
   In the latent content, the patient is saying:

I don't want to talk to my psychiatrist, and I don't like him.
I want to talk to my psychiatrist, and I like him.
I don't want to talk to my therapist, and I don't like him.

T: Yeah, So you go on Monday and fill out the provider change request card and get the injection. If you want to talk about lowering the dose or switching to pills rather than your injection, you can do that. Any number of things you can bring up at the appointment. You mentioned several things to me you might like to discuss.

P: And what if he says no? Like, don't I have a say in what happens to my own body?

In the latent content, the patient is saying:

I think I have a say in what happens to my body.
You don't think I have a say in what happens in therapy.
My psychiatrist doesn't think I have a say in what happens to my body.

T: Sure, of course. If he says no to anything you can ask him to explain why it is a no. You can ask questions and his job is to help you understand why the answer is no. So instead of just hearing no you can get an explanation and have a conversation about it.

P: [Long pause] I really don't like him. [Begins rocking back and forth.]

In the latent content, the patient is saying:

I don't really like you.
I don't really like him.
I really like my psychiatrist.

T: Yeah, yes. And you have something that you want [a specific medication for ADHD] and it is not happening.

P: It hasn't been happening. I've been asking him since June for the same thing and he hasn't done shit about it. And the only reason I'm off all my other meds is because I did that myself. He was not thrilled with me that I did that.

In the latent content, the patient is saying:

You aren't thrilled when I disagree.
My psychiatrist is not thrilled with me when we disagree.
I want to disagree with my psychiatrist.

T: Yup, the two of you disagree on things.

P: A lot of things. I'm a very stubborn person. When I have something in my head it's there and not going away.

T: Yup, I've noticed that.

P: [*Laughter*] When I'm on a mission I'm on a mission.

T: Yup, mmhmm. And that can be a positive, a strength of yours. When you have got something in your focus you are able to really stick to it.

P: Yeah, I wish it worked that way with school.

In the latent content, the patient is saying:

> I wish I could be more stubborn at school.
> I wish I could be more stubborn with you.
> I wish I could be more stubborn with my psychiatrist.

T: So, did you notice that as we were talking about psychiatry and it seemed like you were getting angry, or frustrated, that you started to rock back and forth? Did you notice that connection?

P: [*Shakes her head.*] Mmm-mmm.

T: Yeah so I guess, I did, and I wondered if you did as well. That as some anger came up as we talked about psychiatry that you weren't rocking at all and then started to rock as some anger came up. Did you notice that?

P: I was trying to calm myself down.

T: Right, yeah exactly and trying to calm yourself down because what feelings were you having?

P: A lot of anger. Wanting to go off, again, on him but realizing that there is no point of it.

In the latent content, the patient is saying:

> I realize there is no point expressing anger to my psychiatrist.
> I realize there is no point expressing anger.
> I realize there is no point expressing anger to you.

T: Yeah and you are here with me so you could go off on the psychiatrist, but it's just me who is here. But there was something about anger coming up now and you wanted to calm that down so you started moving, rocking back and forth, which is what you've described to me before when you can't sit still. And it seems like maybe it is happening in this moment, too. Happening right now? Moving a little bit?

P: I've been rocking my feet this whole time.

T: Gotcha, right. But what I noticed was there was a time when even if you were I couldn't see anything. But now I can see more.

P: Oh, okay.

T: So it wasn't just confined to your feet, the rocking was traveling up the body and then I can see it on camera.

P: Oh, okay.

T: And the rocking that I could see started happening as we were talking about psychiatry.

P: Oh, well. I don't like him. That's all I can say. He has rubbed me the wrong way since the beginning. I thought that I was stuck with him.

In the latent content, the patient is saying:

> I think I am stuck with you.
> I think I am stuck.
> I think I am stuck with my psychiatrist.

T: Right, yeah. And so you've told me in the past about being unable to sit still, rocking back and forth, is an issue for you, it bothers you, it makes it hard to get work done. We've talked a little bit about what happens in those moments but not much. But I think what caught my attention today in being with you today was that as I sensed some anger coming up I could also see you were rocking. Which I thought was interesting and something for us to notice together to maybe help you understand yourself a little bit better. These moments where you can't sit still it seems like, at least today here with me, it was a behavior you started to do to manage anger coming up. Kind of gives a reason for the rocking in a new sense, like there is a reason you would rock, right? Like to deal with a feeling?

P: [*Nodding, pause*] Probably, yeah. Like from when I was a kid. Cause my mom was abusive, very abusive to me. And um … I was never allowed to fight back, I had to take it.

In the latent content, the patient is saying:

> I was never allowed to fight back with my mom; I had to take it.
> I cannot fight back with you; I must take it.
> I cannot fight back with the psychiatrist; I must take it.

T: Yeah, so you couldn't fight back, you had to take it.

P: I wasn't allowed to stand up for myself verbally or I got the shit beat out of me.

In the latent content, the patient is saying:

> I'm not allowed to stand up for myself verbally with you.
> I'm not allowed to stand up for myself verbally with my mother.
> I'm not allowed to stand up for myself verbally with my psychiatrist.

Key

*Now you can see how many right answers you found to assess your ability
to listen to latent content. If you missed an answer, go back to the manifest
content and compare it to the latent content in the answer.*

T: So you have an appointment Monday? Your next psychiatry
appointment?

P: Yeah and I don't want to go. I don't know what the point of going is.
What are we going to talk about? I'm going to sit there. For an hour.
Rocking. There's nothing to talk about with him. I really don't like my
psychiatrist.

In the latent content, the patient is saying:

I don't want to talk to my psychiatrist, and I don't like him.
I want to talk to my psychiatrist, and I like him.
I don't want to talk to my therapist, and I don't like him. X

T: Yeah, So you go on Monday and fill out the provider change request
card and get the injection. If you want to talk about lowering the dose
or switching to pills rather than your injection, you can do that. Any
number of things you can bring up at the appointment. You mentioned
several things to me you might like to discuss.

P: And what if he says no? Like, don't I have a say in what happens to my
own body?

In the latent content, the patient is saying:

I think I have a say in what happens to my body.
You don't think I have a say in what happens in therapy. X
My psychiatrist doesn't think I have a say in what happens to my body.

T: Sure, of course. If he says no to anything you can ask him to explain
why it is a no. You can ask questions and his job is to help you understand why the answer is no. So instead of just hearing no you can get an
explanation and have a conversation about it.

P: [*Long pause*] I really don't like him [*Begins rocking back and forth.*]

In the latent content, the patient is saying:

I don't really like you. X
I don't really like him.
I really like my psychiatrist.

T: Yeah, yes. And you have something that you want [a specific medication for ADHD] and it is not happening.

P: It hasn't been happening. I've been asking him since June for the same thing and he hasn't done shit about it. And the only reason I'm off all my other meds is because I did that myself. He was not thrilled with me that I did that.

In the latent content, the patient is saying:

You aren't thrilled when I disagree. X
My psychiatrist is not thrilled with me when we disagree.
I want to disagree with my psychiatrist.

T: Yup, the two of you disagree on things.

P: A lot of things. I'm a very stubborn person. When I have something in my head it's there and not going away.

T: Yup, I've noticed that.

P: [*Laughter*] When I'm on a mission I'm on a mission.

T: Yup, mmhmm. And that can be a positive, a strength of yours. When you have got something in your focus you are able to really stick to it.

P: Yeah, I wish it worked that way with school.

In the latent content, the patient is saying:

I wish I could be more stubborn at school.
I wish I could be more stubborn with you. X
I wish I could be more stubborn with my psychiatrist.

T: So, did you notice that as we were talking about psychiatry and it seemed like you were getting angry, or frustrated, that you started to rock back and forth now? Did you notice that connection?

P: [*Shakes her head.*] Mmm-mmm.

T: Yeah so I guess, I did, and I wondered if you did as well. That as some anger came up as we talked about psychiatry that you weren't rocking at all and then started to rock as some anger came up. Did you notice that?

P: I was trying to calm myself down.

T: Right, yeah exactly and trying to calm yourself down because what feelings were you having?

P: A lot of anger. Wanting to go off, again, on him but realizing that there is no point of it.

In the latent content, the patient is saying:

> I realize there is no point expressing anger to my psychiatrist.
> I realize there is no point expressing anger.
> I realize there is no point expressing anger to you. X

T: Yeah and you are here with me so you could go off on the psychiatrist, but it's just me who is here. But there was something about anger coming up now and you wanted to calm that down so you started moving, rocking back and forth, which is what you've described to me before when you can't sit still. And it seems like maybe it is happening in this moment, too. Happening right now? Moving a little bit?

P: I've been rocking my feet this whole time.

T: Gotcha, right. But what I noticed was there was a time when even if you were I couldn't see anything. But now I can see more.

P: Oh, okay.

T: So it wasn't just confined to your feet the rocking was traveling up the body and then I can see it on camera.

P: Oh, okay.

T: And the rocking that I could see started happening as we were talking about psychiatry.

P: Oh, well. I don't like him. That's all I can say. He has rubbed me the wrong way since the beginning. I thought that I was stuck with him.

In the latent content, the patient is saying:

> I think I am stuck with you. X
> I think I am stuck.
> I think I am stuck with my psychiatrist.

T: Right, yeah. And so you've told me in the past about being unable to sit still, rocking back and forth, is an issue for you, it bothers you, it makes it hard to get work done. We've talked a little bit about what happens in those moments but not much. But I think what caught my attention today in being with you today was that as I sensed some anger coming up I could also see you were rocking. Which I thought was interesting and something for us to notice together to maybe help you understand yourself a little bit better. These moments where you can't sit still it seems like, at least today here with me, it was a behavior you started to do to manage anger coming up. Kind of gives a reason for the rocking in a new sense, like there is a reason you would rock, right? Like to deal with a feeling?

P: [*Nodding, pause*] Probably, yeah. Like from when I was a kid. Cause my mom was abusive, very abusive to me. And um ... I was never allowed to fight back, I had to take it.

In the latent content, the patient is saying:

> I was never allowed to fight back with my mom; I had to take it.
> I cannot fight back with you; I must take it. X
> I cannot fight back with the psychiatrist; I must take it.

T: Yeah, so you couldn't fight back, you had to take it.
P: I wasn't allowed to stand up for myself verbally or I got the shit beat out of me.

In the latent content, the patient is saying:

> I'm not allowed to stand up for myself verbally with you. X
> I'm not allowed to stand up for myself verbally with my mother.
> I'm not allowed to stand up for myself verbally with my psychiatrist.

Appendix B

A Deliberate Practice Skill-Building Exercise for Learning Procedural Knowledge

Skill-Building Exercise: Offering Non-Problems Rather than Real Problems

Fifty percent of patients leave therapy before receiving the full benefit. And if patients don't improve within the first seven sessions, they aren't likely to get better (Wierzbidki & Pekorik, 1993). Why don't they improve? They don't form an effective therapeutic alliance. In any good working alliance, partners agree on what they will do and why they will do it (Bordin, 1994). The problem is the reason the patient comes to therapy. That's why both the therapist and patient must agree on the problem the patient wants to resolve.

When patients have trouble declaring a problem to work on, they offer a non-problem instead of a real problem. For instance, the patient might present something that sounds like a problem for someone else but not for the patient. Do not explore any issue, no matter how severe, if the patient does not regard it as a problem. If she does not consider it a problem, she is not motivated to explore it. Here's an example:

T: What is the problem you would like me to help you with?
P: I'm living with my husband, but he's just a placeholder for now until I leave.
T: Is that a problem you would like me to help you with?
P: No. I'm fine with it.
T: Okay. Since that's not a problem for you, what is the problem you would like me to help you with?

Do not argue with the patient. In therapy, we explore what *she* thinks is a problem, not what *we* think is a problem. If she regards something as not a problem, we have no right to explore it. In fact, our respect for her wish not to explore an issue often mobilizes her desire to explore it.

When patients present a non-problem, you can respond by saying, "It's not clear how that is a problem for you. So what is the problem you'd like me to help you with?" If they maintain that everything is fine, you can respond, "Great! Yet if everything were fine, you wouldn't be here. So I wonder: what the problem is you would like me to help you with?"

Playing the patient, read the following to your partner who is in the therapist role:

I will play a patient who responds with non-problems. Block my non-problem and return the focus to an internal problem. After you answer, I'll give you the recommended answer. Don't worry if your words are not identical to those in the book. As long as you block the avoidance strategy and return the focus to the problem, your answer will be fine. The goal here is not to repeat the words in the book but to learn the principle guiding those words: block a non-problem and return to the focus on an internal problem.

Here you will learn how to block misalliance behaviors to promote a therapeutic alliance. Now we will begin the role-play exercise. Ask me, "What is the problem you want me to help you with?"

[Note to the reader: in the following skill-building exercise, the responses marked Pt: are stated by the student in the patient role. Her partner, in the therapist role, must figure out how to respond. And the text in italics that follows is a suggested response. Through this structured role-play exercise, students learn a skill by doing it together. The partner who plays the patient has the script. The student who plays the therapist does not have the script. That way she must think on her feet and generate interventions, just like she would have to in the therapy room with her patients.]

P: My kids are doing well, my job is great, and overall everything is going fine.

[T: *That's wonderful. But if everything were going wonderfully, you wouldn't be here. So what is the problem you'd like me to help you with?*]

P: I want my kids to do better in school, and I was hoping you could help me help them. [T: *I hear that your kids have a problem at school. But it's not clear how that is an internal problem for you. So what is your problem that you would like me to help you with?*]

P: I don't know.

[T: *And yet, you are here. So what is the problem you would like me to help you with?*]

P: My wife and I have been in couples therapy, and the couples therapist recommended I see you since the literature shows, she said, that couples therapy plus individual therapy is the best combination.

[T: *"This is what your therapist said, but it is not clear what the problem is you would like me to help you with. What is the problem you would like me to help you with?"*]

P: The human resources people also recommended I see you. I'm a high-level executive. I'm very successful and good at what I do. I'm the person they send in to close the deal because they know I'm very good with people.

[T: *"That's great, so can you be more specific about what you want me to help you with?"*]

P: My ex-girlfriend said I should see a therapist. I told her about the affair I'm having, and she really reamed me out over that. [*Rolls his eyes.*] She thinks I shouldn't be unfaithful to my wife. She's probably right. But you know I've been having affairs in my marriage for twenty years. It's a great way to be sexually satisfied, and women are always hitting on me, eager to hop into bed. Who am I to say no?

[T: *"You say it's a problem for your ex-girlfriend, but it's not clear how this is a problem for you. What is the problem you would like me to help you with?"*]

P: I'm an adult child of an alcoholic, and I've been reading a lot of books about that. My father and mother were both drinkers. And, from what I've read, it's clear that what parents do to you influences your adult life.

[T: *"Before we go into your history, could you be more specific about what your problem is today that you want me to help you with?"*]

P: I wondered if my wife had been having an affair. She denied it and denied it. But then, about two weeks ago, before I called you, she told me she had had an affair. So anyway, we have talked about it and thought the most logical solution would be for us to divorce. She would take the kids and move to New Jersey, and I would stay here and have the kids with me two months a year.

[T: *"You mention the affairs and the solution of divorce and childcare arrangements. But it's still not clear how this is an internal emotional problem for you. What is the problem you want me to help you with?"*]

P: I'm not sure what to work on. I hadn't thought of anything. I suppose we could talk about my drug use. But to be honest, it's not a big deal for me.

[T: *"Since the drug use is not a big deal for you, what is the internal problem you would like me to help you with?"*]

P: My wife is very controlling. We have been in marital therapy for years but with no result. She is still controlling. I have tried talking to her about it, but it doesn't do any good.

[T: *"You have described your wife, but it's not clear how this is an internal emotional problem for you. Could you be more specific about the internal emotional problem you would like me to help you with?"*]

P: She said that if I don't start treating her better, I have to move out.

[T: *"And is this pattern with your wife the problem you want us to work on together?"*]

P: [*sigh*] Yes, because I don't want to lose her and the kids.

When patients avoid declaring a problem quickly, they don't sit around thinking, "Hmm, which avoidance strategy could I use?" They avoid automatically. They don't even know they are avoiding. When you block these strategies as rapidly as they come up, the patient will soon offer a problem and get the help he needs.

Let's do the exercise again. Whenever you intervene, I, as the patient, will go immediately to the next patient statement. Let's make this exercise feel like a real session. We won't stop for chitchat. We'll go straight through, so that you get the experience of processing and intervening more quickly. We'll repeat it several times. After you master this exercise, we'll shift roles so I can master it too. As long as you block the avoidance strategy and return the focus to the problem, your answer will be fine. The goal here is not to repeat the words in the book but to learn the principle guiding those words: block a non-problem and return to the focus on an internal problem.

Questions to ask each other to strengthen your skills: After doing this skill-building exercise, how would you differentiate an internal emotional problem from a non-problem? How does recognizing a non-problem change your understanding of the patient's conflict about depending? How does recognizing a non-problem change your understanding about what we mean by a therapeutic focus? What did you learn through the therapist's clear therapeutic focus when you were in the patient role? What did you experience when your partner blocked avoidance strategies? What advice might you give your partner? What is it like for you to see avoidance strategies that the patient cannot see? How does this change your understanding of the patient when you see how automatic strategies can occur outside the patient's awareness?

Commentary on the Skill-Building Exercise

A skill-building exercise focuses on only one skill across numerous patient responses. It begins with a brief discussion of the theory of that technique. Then the skill-building exercise helps students put theory into practice. Students divide up into pairs. First, one student plays the therapist, and the other plays the patient. The "therapist" does not read from the exercise because she would only learn to read. Instead, she must figure out how to respond without the script—just as she would have to in therapy. From her struggle, she learns how to intervene. The student in the patient role learns from experience how this skill feels to the patient. She identifies with the patient and experiences the world from that point of view. Thus, that student develops a theory of mind of the patient through role-play. After they go through the entire exercise, the two students switch roles. The former therapist is now in the patient role. And the former patient is in the therapist role. Then they repeat the exercise. And they repeat the exercise, changing roles until each of them has mastered that skill.

[Exercise taken from Frederickson, 2023.]

References

Bordin, E. S. (1994). Theory and research on the therapeutic working alliance: New directions. In A. Horvath & L. Greenberg (Eds.), *The working alliance: Theory, research, and practice* (pp. 13–37). New York: Wiley.

Frederickson, J. (2023). *Healing through relating: A skill-building book for therapists*. Kensington, Md.: Seven Leaves Press.

Wierzbidki, M., & Pekorik, G. (1993). A meta-analysis of psychotherapy drop out. *Professional Psychology: Research and Practice, 24,* 190–195.

Index

Note: Page numbers in *italics* refer to figures. Numbers in **bold** indicate tables.